PHYSICAL DIAGNOSIS

FOR SURGICAL STUDENTS

Syed Asif Razvi, MD

Order this book online at www.trafford.com
or email orders@trafford.com

Most Trafford titles are also available at major online book retailers.

Printed in the United States of America.

ISBN: 978-1-4669-7135-6 (sc)
ISBN: 978-1-4669-7137-0 (hc)
ISBN: 978-1-4669-7136-3 (e)

Library of Congress Control Number: 2012922773

Trafford rev. 12/03/2012

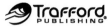 www.trafford.com

North America & international
toll-free: 1 888 232 4444 (USA & Canada)
phone: 250 383 6864 ♦ fax: 812 355 4082

This book is dedicated to my brother, the
late Syed Ahsan Razvi, MD.
"A great clinician and a cardiologist loved and
respected by thousands of his patients"

CONTENTS

INTRODUCTION

Physical diagnosis is rapidly becoming a forgotten art in the practice of modern-day medicine. Dependence on ancillary tools (lab work and imaging) for making a diagnosis has reached near-addiction levels. It is lack of knowledge of physical diagnosis that results in physicians ordering a lot of unnecessary tests. Uncertainty about the physician's ability to make a diagnosis by physical examination not only adds to poor quality of care, but also significantly increases the cost of care. Lack of confidence in making the diagnosis increases fear of litigation and makes the physician order a lot more tests than what are required, thus contributing to the escalating cost of medical care today.

Experienced physicians with expertise in physical diagnosis and willingness to teach this art are few and far between. There are no practical handbooks of surgical physical diagnosis for medical students or young surgeons in training that can be conveniently carried with them for ready reference. The purpose of this work is to provide such a guide for the medical students during their surgical clerkship and also make it useful for PGY (Post Graduate Year) 1 surgical residents.

This handbook will use the classic tools of physical diagnosis, which include inspection, palpation, percussion, and auscultation. Appropriate examples will depict the correct methods of examination. The differential diagnosis will be looked upon in the light of conditions being congenital or acquired, and the acquired conditions could be traumatic, inflammatory, or neoplastic.

Accuracy in arriving at a diagnosis is dependent on the correlation between a thorough history taking and the physical findings. It takes an effort to learn to develop proper listening skills to take a good history. It is not uncommon for a patient who is a good historian to give away the diagnosis if the medical student or a house officer on the other end has been listening and paying attention to what is being said.

Some suggestions for proper history taking relative to the chief complaint will be included in this text.

HISTORY TAKING

H istory taking is an integral part of physical diagnosis, and unfortunately, there is not enough stress on its importance and methodology. As America has increasingly become a melting pot of diverse cultures and ethnicities, the art of extracting pertinent and useful information from patients has become challenging. Some patients love to talk and blurt out a lot of unnecessary information that may not have anything to do with their chief complaint, whereas others will not open up to every physician and hold back important information. It is important to know what kinds of leading questions need to be asked to get the necessary information. For example, a patient with a complaint of recurrent gastrointestinal bleeding might not be able to shed any light on the magnitude of the previous bleed; however, if asked about the number of blood transfusions received, this patient might know the answer.

It is a good idea to adopt a system or a method of history taking and stick to it so one does not forget any important steps. The usual and customary method is to start with the *chief complaint*, followed in sequence with the *history of present illness*, *past medical history*, *past surgical history*, *social history*, *current medications*, and *known drug allergies*. Following the sequence or method is not as much of a problem as obtaining accurate information. The first student or resident recording information on a newly admitted patient has a lot of responsibility on his/her shoulders. Unfortunately, it is common practice for students or residents to copy information from the old records during subsequent hospital admissions. So any incorrect information is likely to get recorded year after year without being corrected until a compulsive or a thorough student actually talks with the patient or the family to verify the facts.

One of the most important steps in history taking is to gain the patient's confidence first. Many psychologists have studied the doctor-patient interactions and concluded that many patients are astute observers and they are studying the doctor while the doctor is talking to them. They prefer that the person talking with them make eye contact. It is preferable to sit down by the bedside to make the patient believe that you have all the time in the world and you have their undivided attention. Never stand in the doorway while speaking, and avoid putting your hands in your pockets.

It is beyond the scope of this book to elaborate on every symptom of surgical disease, but an attempt is made to offer some practical hints on the most common surgical symptoms.

PAIN

1. Onset of pain: Whether sudden or gradual helps one decide if the problem was acute or chronic.
2. Character of pain: Sharp pain may be indicative, for example, of a perforated viscus, whereas dull pain will suggest an inflammatory process. A stabbing pain is seen in a dissecting aneurysm, and a colicky pain in bowel obstruction or kidney

stone. As each one of these characters of pain are suggestive of a diagnosis, it is important to document this finding. Pain is now expressed on a scale of one to ten, with ten being the most severe.

3. Radiation of pain: A right upper-quadrant pain radiating around to the back is typical of biliary colic. An epigastric pain radiating straight through to the back is often seen in pancreatitis. It is important to know some unusual patterns of radiation in some situations; for example, pancreatitis may present with pain in the right lower quadrant, or gall bladder disease may present with chest pain.

4. Exacerbation or relief of pain: For example, pain from a muscle tear will be exacerbated with walking or exercise, whereas pain from a duodenal ulcer will be relieved by eating.

5. Associated symptoms: Association of nausea and vomiting and diarrhea and constipation, and determination of whether these symptoms preceded or followed the onset of pain are important to know.

6. Relationship to food: Pain following a fatty meal is suggestive of gall bladder disease; pain immediately following eating may suggest gastritis or gastric ulcer. Sometimes the type of food eaten and the onset of pain give one a clue to the possible etiology. An example of this would be eating chicken and developing pain several hours afterward may be secondary to chicken-bone perforation of the small intestine.

MASS, SWELLING, OR A LUMP

1. Duration: It is very helpful to know how long the mass has been present. Duration generally relates directly to the acuteness or chronicity of the mass. For example, a short-duration mass may be an inflammatory process as opposed to a lipoma that may have been present for a long time.

2. Location: It is extremely important to be precise with the description of location, as this in itself will be an important clue to differential diagnosis. For a simple example, a midline neck mass that moves with swallowing is a thyroid mass.

3. Growth and rate of growth: Slow growth or no growth is generally indicative of a benign process. Rapid rate of growth may be seen in an inflammatory process or a malignancy.

4. Pain and tenderness: Pain and tenderness are often associated with an inflammatory process or closeness of the mass to a sensory nerve.

5. Consistency: The lump may be solid or cystic. Cystic masses tend to be benign, except in rare cases where a tumor may have undergone cystic degeneration.

6. Transillumination: Cystic masses that transilluminate are reassuring as they are often benign. An example would be a cystic hygroma or a hydrocele.

7. Overlying skin: Erythematous changes in the overlying skin that blanch are suggestive of an inflammatory process. Light-brown spots on the overlying skin (café au lait)

are seen in neurofibromas. Presence of a small dark dot (punctum) in the center of the overlying skin is diagnostic of a sebaceous cyst.

8. Mobility: It is important to determine if the mass is freely movable in the tissue underneath the skin. A mass that is fixed may be fixed because of its attachment to the skin (lipoma) or invasion of deeper tissues (malignancy). A mass that moves only in one direction is generally because it is arising in or from a muscle.

9. Palpability of the mass: A mass that becomes more prominent by contraction of a muscle underneath is located superficial to that muscle. If the mass becomes less prominent or less palpable with the contraction of the muscle, it is located deeper to the muscle. A mass that stays the same with the contraction of the muscle is located in the muscle. This determination is important when you are evaluating an abdominal mass to see if it is in the wall of the abdomen or deeper.

10. Pulsatility of the mass: If a mass is pulsatile, it is important to determine if the pulsations are transmitted or expansile. Transmitted pulsations only mean that the mass is located on top of an artery, whereas expansile pulsations are present only in aneurysms.

11. Borders: Well-defined or well-circumscribed borders are again indicative of a benign process—for example, a lipoma, fibroma, etc.

12. Reducibility of the mass: A reducible mass in an appropriate location will be diagnostic of a hernia.

ULCER

1. Location: A common presenting symptom of a surgical patient is a lower-extremity ulcer; however ulcers may be present anywhere on the body. As lower-extremity ulcers are the more common presenting symptom, our focus will primarily be on that. It is very important to be specific with the location of the ulcer on the lower extremity. Venous ulcers (probably the most common) tend to be located on the medial aspect of the leg in the distal third of the leg (gaiter area), where there is increased venous pressure from an incompetent communicating or perforating vein, Whereas arterial ulcers tend to occur on pressure points like the malleoli, some arterial ulcers may be located at the tips of toes or in between the toes. Ulcers secondary to trauma may be located at the site of injury and could be anywhere on the lower extremity.

2. Pain: Absence of pain should immediately draw attention to the fact that this may be secondary to neuropathy. One of the more common neuropathies is a complication of diabetes. The examiner should be aware, of course, that there are other etiologies for lack of sensation in the lower extremity.

3. Any change since onset: An ulcer that has a history of improvement from time to time but is persistent is more consistent with a chronic venous ulcer. An ulcer that has progressively gotten worse with absolutely no signs of healing will be typical of an arterial ulcer. A traumatic ulcer that was getting better and then suddenly became

more painful and looked worse could be an indication of secondary infection.

4. Bleeding: When the patient gives a history of finding blood stains on the dressing (as commonly seen from granulation tissue), it needs clear distinction from actual hemorrhage from the ulcer. A venous ulcer with a spontaneous rupture of a vein can spurt blood like an artery and can be very alarming and scary for the patient.

5. Systemic diseases: An ulcer may be the cutaneous manifestation of certain systemic diseases. For example, tuberculosis, lupus, parasitic infections, and hypertension, to name a few.

BLEEDING

Bleeding from the GI tract is a relatively common presenting symptom. GI bleeding may present itself as an acute massive hemorrhage from the upper or lower GI tract, chronic blood loss usually from the lower GI tract, or subtle blood loss presenting with symptoms of chronic blood-loss anemia.

Acute Upper-GI Bleed

When someone presents to the emergency treatment center with a history of having vomited blood, there are many important historical facts to inquire about:

1. Quantity: How much blood was brought up? Give examples like a spoonful to basinful. Is this a first episode of bleeding, or have there been previous episodes of bleeding? If there is

history of bleeding in the past, find out how many times the patient bled and if the patient ever required hospitalization for any of those bleeds. A history of hospitalization or need for transfusion gives you an idea about the magnitude of the bleed in the past. For the presenting symptom of bleeding, hemodynamic instability generally points toward the magnitude of the bleed.

2. Associated symptoms like nausea before vomiting or severe retching before vomiting. History of severe retching before vomiting blood makes one suspect a Mallory-Weiss tear of the GE junction.

3. Any history of binge drinking problem. A positive history leads one to consider acute alcoholic gastritis.

4. Past medical history: Is there any past history of peptic ulcer disease or esophageal varices. It is important to remember that even with a history of esophageal varices, a third of acute upper-GI hemorrhage is secondary to a peptic ulcer in patients with varices. If the patient had a previous bleed, ask them if they were ever told they had an AVM. It is also important to know that if the patient ever had an abdominal aortic aneurysm repaired as an aortoduodenal fistula, it is often a fatal long-term complication of an open repair of AAA.

5. Rectal bleeding: One has to be aware of the fact that a significant upper-GI bleed may present with only rectal bleeding and no history of vomiting blood. This is why when you are presented with a patient with significant rectal bleeding, it is essential to put down a nasogastric tube to rule out an upper-GI source of bleeding.

Acute Lower-GI Bleed

The most common cause of rectal bleeding in an adult is diverticulosis of the colon. On the other hand, the most common cause of finding blood in a child's diaper is an anal fissure. We would go through a similar line of questioning for the lower-GI bleeding as we did for the upper, with some minor variations.

1. Quantity: Besides diverticulosis coli causing massive lower-GI bleeding, an AVM also presents with a significant rectal bleeding as well. In addition to other things mentioned for the upper-GI bleed, it is important to find out if there has been a history of hemorrhoids. It is sometimes embarrassing to put the patient through all kinds of workup and miss an easily diagnosed hemorrhoidal bleed. Passage of clots indicates the severity of the bleed.

2. Change in bowels: Either change in the bowel habit going from normal to constipation or change in the caliber of stool may be pertinent to suspect a colonic neoplasm. Sometimes diarrhea may be associated with a villous adenoma, or it may be spurious diarrhea related to colonic obstruction. Lower-GI bleeding from a colonic or rectal neoplasm is more likely to be chronic rather than acute.

3. Presence of anal fissure may be cause of an acute lower-GI bleed; however, this is never severe.

4. A less frequent cause of acute lower-GI bleed may be erosion of a prolapsing rectum or a stercoral ulcer.

5. Presence of abdominal pain and distention associated with a rectal bleed may be due to an intussusception.

Indigestion

Symptoms associated with diseases of the gall bladder, stomach (peptic ulcer disease), and esophagogastric junction (hiatus hernia) are generally overlapping symptoms and sometimes difficult to separate one from the other.

1. Abdominal distension and a bloated feeling after eating, particularly fried or fatty food is suggestive of gall bladder dyspepsia and is often associated with biliary tract disease. However, some patients with a peptic ulcer or gastroesophageal reflux disease (GERD) may have similar symptoms. Most patients are not very clear with the description of exactly what they feel, and this is what causes confusion.

2. Excessive eructation (burping): When patients feel like the food they ate is just sitting in the pit of their stomachs and not moving, they think that burping will be advantageous. What the patients do not appreciate is that eructation causes them to swallow more air, which makes the discomfort worse.

3. Malabsorption: Chronic pancreatitis in an adult will cause diarrhea, abdominal pain, and passage of excessive fats and undigested food in their stools. In children, this may be seen with sprue or celiac disease.

It is beyond the scope of this book to cover every symptom a patient may present with. A few common examples were picked to give the student of surgery an idea about the line of thought process and questioning when they are evaluating a patient to arrive at a bedside diagnosis. As mentioned earlier in the introduction to this book today's student relies heavily on the ancillary tests and therefore has gotten away from a logical thought process to put the pieces of the puzzle together from a good history and physical examination to arrive at a bedside diagnosis.

PHYSICAL EXAMINATION
GENERAL PRINCIPLES

The age-old teaching of conducting a physical examination in a systematic way allows one to be thorough and less likely to miss important findings. The well-established four steps of inspection, palpation, percussion, and auscultation still hold true in the majority of cases. Once a complete history is taken and you are formulating a differential diagnosis in your mind, each of these steps of physical examination should get you closer to your bedside diagnosis. We will now address the general principles of each one of these steps so the student should be able to apply these to any system that is being examined.

Inspection

It is astonishing how much information can be obtained by just looking at the patient. While you are taking the history, you could be inspecting the patient at the same time. It is important to gain the patient's confidence while you are taking the history and inspecting him/her at the same time. This was addressed earlier in the history taking. The power of observation can be very rewarding.

Note if the patient is lying comfortably in bed or appears restless. Also make note of the posturing, whether the patient is turned to one side, holding on to a certain part of his/her body, has one or both legs drawn up into the abdomen, is grimacing with pain, or is sitting up in bed with the feet dangling. Remember that every one of these postures means something. For example, a patient lying down with the legs drawn up might have an acute abdominal process and finds comfort in that position. The individual postures will be dealt with at their appropriate places in this manuscript.

Pale appearance of a patient is indicative of anemia, and sunken eyeballs and wrinkled skin generally mean dehydration. Sometimes jaundice will present with a subtle change in the skin color or color of sclera.

On the other hand, an obviously jaundiced patient with scratch marks on the skin is suggestive of a high bilirubin, causing severe itch.

One of the cardinal rules of a good physical examination is to examine the patient from head to feet. So there should be no reluctance in asking the patient to undress to make it easy for you to examine the entire body surface, both front and back. Always remember to protect the patient's modesty and only expose the area that is being examined. Look for any skin abnormality, lumps and bumps, any pigmentation or pigmented lesions, any scars of previous wounds or operations, any visible pulsations, and any bony deformities. In addition, look for any neurologic abnormalities like a drooping eyelid, nystagmus, tremor, wrist drop, or foot drop. Some endocrine pathologies might be obvious on inspection alone—for example, an exophthalmic goiter, acromegalic facies, or a cushiongoid face.

A patient with COPD (chronic obstructive pulmonary disease) is generally obvious with the accessory muscles of respiration at work. A congestive heart failure patient with jugular venous distension and shortness of breath and peripheral edema can be spotted even from a distance.

These are just a few examples of the hundreds of diagnoses that can be made just on inspecting the patients.

Palpation

There is no more sensitive diagnostic tool than the palpating fingers of a knowledgeable examining physician. History has taught us that in ancient times, physicians would just palpate the pulse of a patient and come up with a possible diagnosis. Centuries later, with all the modern diagnostic imaging and technology and having spent millions of dollars, sometimes one wonders if we are really that much better off than those brilliant physicians of the past.

Palpation not only offers additional information to inspection, but it is also believed by many to have some psychological benefits from a patient's perspective. Touching to examine the patients may have the added benefit of the perception of a healing hand touching the patient or comforting the patient and often making the patient believe that you have a genuine interest in his/her well-being.

It is important to warm up your hands before you lay them on the patient, another sign of compassion and caring.

Touching the patient tells you whether they are normothermic, their skin is dry or moist, and/or they are hypersensitive. Checking the pulse gives you a crude examination of the heart by giving you the rate and/or irregularities.

Examination of a lump can tell you about its mobility or fixation or tenderness and pulsatility. Palpation of the abdomen can reveal important information on organomegaly, tenderness, or rebound tenderness.

Techniques of palpation of the abdomen, checking for fluctuance in a swelling, eliciting a Homans' sign, and others, will be detailed in their appropriate chapters.

Percussion

Probably the least practiced method of evaluation. This method of evaluation is most useful in examination of an abdomen. Some of the examples are checking for rebound tenderness by percussion technique, outlining an abdominal mass, checking for absence of liver dullness, documenting a distended urinary bladder, and presence of bowel in a hernia. One can also percuss for the level of a pleural effusion or borders of an enlarged heart.

Though not classic percussion, some examples of tapping to elicit signs are Chvostek's sign for hypocalcemia and Tinel's sign for nerve regeneration.

When one is evaluating a mass anywhere, percussion may differentiate a gas-filled mass from a fluid-filled mass in addition to establishing tenderness.

Auscultation

I believe it is the most common method of examination utilized by physicians and other paramedical personnel. From using the stethoscope for listening to the arteries for bruits to listening for abnormalities of breath sounds, heart sounds, and bowel sounds, auscultation can serve as a very important diagnostic tool. A few pointers will be mentioned here in connection with its utility in examination of the various systems.

Examination of carotid arteries for presence of a bruit can be tricky for two reasons. First and foremost, one needs to know the best location for listening for a carotid bruit, as it is a common mistake to think of a transmitted murmur to be a bruit. The ideal spot to listen for carotid bruit is at its bifurcation, which is anatomically marked by the level of the thyroid cartilage. If you listen at the level of the thyroid cartilage directly over the carotid, a bruit should be loudest at that location. As you move away from that location, the intensity of the sound will diminish. If the intensity of the sound is unchanged from suprasternal notch to the angle of the jaw, it is likely a transmitted heart murmur. Sometimes this evaluation is difficult as the change in intensity may be subtle.

Auscultation of the chest for breath sounds and heart sounds is an extremely valuable examination. The examiner is able to establish presence or absence of breath sounds over different lung fields, presence of normal breath sounds versus bronchial breathing, presence of wheezing indicating bronchospasm, or that breath sounds may be distant.

Listening to heart sounds gives information about the heart rhythm, heart murmurs and their character, a clicking sound of a prosthetic heart valve, or a friction sound of a pericardial rub.

A stethoscope can be used very effectively to palpate an abdomen while listening. When a patient presents with abdominal pain and you approach them with your hand for palpation, the patient will voluntarily guard the abdomen with concern that you will hurt them. As opposed to that, if you approach them with your stethoscope and palpate their abdomen pretending to listen, the patient will stay more relaxed. It is always a good idea to auscultate before you palpate the abdomen, particularly listening for bowel sounds, because the act of palpation can sometimes mechanically stimulate the bowel and misguide you with a few bowel sounds in an otherwise silent abdomen. In addition to determination of presence or absence of bowel sounds, it is important to note whether the sounds are low pitched, high pitched, hypo- or hyperactive, to the point of being audible to bystanders (borborygmi).

What is described above is the basic knowledge every student of surgery is expected to know and learn about.

EXAMINATION OF SKIN AND SOFT TISSUES

E xamination of skin and soft tissues will be described again in the standard method of starting with inspection and ending with auscultation.

Inspection

A good student of surgery has to have keen observation skills. The first thing that is obvious to the examiner is the color of skin.

Pallor: Generally indicative of anemia. Patients of certain ethnicity may give the appearance of pallor without being anemic. A quick examination of the mucosal surfaces should settle that definitively.

Erythema: Redness of the skin is one of the most common observations. Some frequently seen problems causing redness include first-degree burn (or a sunburn), cellulites, or a skin rash.

Cyanosis: Usually means decreased perfusion of skin, resulting in a bluish-purplish hue to the color of skin. This is seen in many conditions—for example, a patient with chronic obstructive pulmonary disease (COPD) or someone with peripheral vascular disease (PVD). The important thing here is making the observation and having the ability to come up with this finding, as in some cases, this may be a very subtle change. One should realize that cyanosis may be present because of local factors or systemic factors. A perfect example of local factors would be cyanosis of a part of the body secondary to exposure to severe cold. As mentioned earlier, systemic factors could be cardiac or pulmonary.

Jaundice: Yellowish discoloration of the skin may be subtle or obvious depending on the level of jaundice. Along with the skin, there is yellowish discoloration of the _ucces and mucous membranes as well. Clinical jaundice is usually not detectable until the serum direct bilirubin gets above 2.5 mg. Remember that some skin complexions make it harder to appreciate the color change.

Flushing: Patients who appear flushed may be having a high fever, may be having an allergic reaction to something, may be having a hypertensive episode, or may be having a skin manifestation of a systemic syndrome.

Bruising: Skin will be bruised as a result of trauma, spontaneous bleeding from a bleeding disorder, or use of antiplatelet agents or anticoagulation. It is important to get a detailed history, including family history, if a hematologic disorder is suspected.

Petechiae: Small dot-like capillary hemorrhage in the skin may be a manifestation of numerous medical diseases; however, from a surgeon's point of view, the important causes to remember are thrombocytopenia, peripheral emboli, and trauma.

Dimpling or puckering of skin: Commonly seen as manifestation of scarring, may represent a serious underlying problem like a tumor.

Peau d'orange: A change seen in the skin of a female breast when the skin appears to look like orange peel. This is a classic presentation of an *inflammatory carcinoma of breast*.

Black skin: Black skin is an obvious sign of necrosis or gangrene from any cause.

Skin blisters: There are several blistering diseases in the field of dermatology beyond the scope of this book; however, some blisters a surgeon should be aware of are blisters secondary to edema, blisters from an insect bite, and of course, burns.

Skin pigmentation: Faint pigmentation may be present over underlying *neurofibromatosis* (café au lait spots), heavy brown pigmentation seen with hemosiderin deposits in chronic venous stasis, or the peculiar bronze discoloration seen with *hemochromatosis*. When examining pigmented lesions, it is important to note how long they have been present and if there has been any change. With a rising incidence of *melanoma,* it is essential to do a complete examination of the skin, particularly skin of the back and skin of the back of the legs, two locations often ignored during routine examinations. Changes in color of a mole or appearance of ulceration are highly significant.

Abnormal vasculature: Venous or arteriovenous malformations may be quite evident on inspection alone. Presence of prominent veins in the skin of various parts of the body carries special significance. For instance, presence of a cluster of veins around the umbilicus (caput medusae) is a hallmark of *portal hypertension*.

Visible mass: Make note of any visible masses. Special attention should be paid to the skin overlying the mass. Observe any pulsatility to the mass and any peculiarity about its size and shape.

In addition to what is mentioned above, every physical exam should include a thorough survey of the skin of the entire body, making a note of moles, raised skin lesions, or any breach in the continuity of skin like a laceration or ulcer.

Palpation

Following up on visual inspection of skin and soft tissues, the tactile sensation of the examiner can be greatly supportive of the visual findings. The various findings that can be elicited by palpation are as follows:

Skin temperature: Skin temperature is warm in patients with fever or flushed appearance from vasodilatation. A patient in circulatory collapse may have cold, moist skin. A recently revascularized limb will have warmer skin temperature whereas a patient with vasomotor disorder will have cool skin temperature—for example, Raynaud's disease.

Skin turgor: Skin turgor is generally a good indicator of the status of hydration of a patient. A loss of skin turgor is commonly seen in patients with severe fluid loss due to poor intake, severe diarrhea, or vomiting.

Hypersensitivity: Skin hypersensitivity may be associated with certain inflammatory conditions within the abdomen like acute appendicitis (Sherren's triangle).

Swelling: The very first step is to determine if the swelling is of the skin or a mass underneath the skin. The skin may be swollen for many reasons, of which skin edema is a common cause. Skin edema may be secondary to trauma, infection, fluid accumulation, or a neoplasm. If there is a mass palpable underneath the skin, it

21

is important to note several following features that help make a diagnosis.

Mobility: Is the mass freely movable under the skin, or is there a skin attachment? A sebaceous cyst will be attached to the skin where a punctum (duct opening) may be visible.

Direction of mobility determines its attachment to a muscle or tendon when it will move only in one direction.

Consistency: Generally described as soft, firm, or hard; carries a different meaning with each descriptive term. Softness is attributed to cystic structures or fatty masses. Firmness is associated with solid masses that are mostly benign but could have early malignant changes. Hardness is almost always suspicious of malignancy, though some masses containing calcification may feel hard as well. One should be aware that some hematomas feel very hard, but a hematoma may be associated some ecchymosis or discoloration of the overlying skin.

Tenderness: A tender mass underneath the skin is usually indicative of one of two things. Firstly, it may be an inflammatory or infected swelling that tends to be tender to palpation. Secondly, a mass sitting on top of a cutaneous nerve or a mass arising from a nerve itself will be tender to palpation.

Fluctuance: Fluctuance is usually a sign of a cyst or an abscess. Fluctuance is tested by placing the index finger and thumb on either side of the swelling and applying pressure on the center of the mass with the other index finger. If this maneuver separates the thumb and index finger, it will be a positive sign for fluctuance. The finger applying pressure in the center of the mass will also experience a softness to the center of the swelling.

Location of the swelling: Here we will talk about determination of the depth of the mass. For example, if there is swelling on the abdomen, it is important to know whether this swelling is in the abdominal wall or is intra-abdominal. To establish this, ask the patient to tense up the muscles in the area of the swelling. If the swelling becomes more prominent, it will mean that the swelling is located in the abdominal wall and is most likely superficial to the muscles. If the swelling does not change at all with the tensing up of the muscles, it is still located in the abdominal wall and probably in the muscle layer. However, if the swelling disappears with the muscle contraction, it is located in the abdominal cavity and is determined to be intra-abdominal.

Pulsatility: A pulsatile swelling under the skin may be secondary to a mass overlying an artery or an aneurysm of the artery itself. To establish which it is, one checks to see if the pulsations are transmitted or if they are expansile. If two fingers placed on a pulsatile swelling separated from each other, they will be observed to move up and down if the pulsations are transmitted; however, if the pulsations are expansile, the fingers will go not only up and down but also apart with each pulsation.

Edge: Attempt to palpate the border or the edge of the swelling. If the edge is palpable and feels ropy under the palpating finger, the swelling is likely to be a *lipoma*. A rounded edge is usually palpated in a cyst or an encapsulated mass.

Reducibility: For a swelling or a mass to be reducible, it has to communicate with a body cavity. Examples would be an abdominal hernia, a synovial cyst, a meningomyelocele, etc. Obviously, the location of the swelling determines its etiology.

Overlying skin: Attachment to the overlying skin is not necessarily a bad sign. As mentioned earlier, a sebaceous cyst tends to be attached to the skin, and so do some lipomas. Ulceration of skin overlying a mass is highly suspicious of the mass being a neoplasm.

Percussion

In examination of skin and soft tissues, percussion has very limited application. Percussion may be of value in determining if the swelling or mass being percussed contains air. Presence of air can be equated to presence of bowel and is therefore an important finding in evaluating a nonreducible hernia, for example.

A rare instance of percussion of air in an abscess is indicative of an anaerobic infection with gas-producing organisms, which may be highly significant.

Percussion technique may be used sometimes to elicit tenderness in a mass or swelling as it tends to minimize the patient's fear of an examining hand.

Auscultation

Like percussion, auscultation also has limited value in examination of skin and soft tissues. As in the case of a hernia, if you percuss bowel in a swelling, hearing bowel sounds on auscultation will confirm the presence of bowel in the hernia sac. Auscultation of a bruit over a swelling will indicate that swelling to be of vascular etiology.

HEAD AND NECK

T he head and neck area will be dealt with by paying special
attention to problems encountered by a student of surgery.
There are some areas that are in a gray zone, and a clear separation
between medical and surgical pathologies will be difficult.

HEAD

Examination of the head will be divided into the scalp and face,
the oral cavity including the tongue and tonsils, and the parotid
region.

Scalp and Face

One of the most common problems that are seen surgically are
single or multiple bumps or swellings of the scalp. These swellings
are freely movable underneath the skin, and they are often nontender.
These are *pilar cysts*, which arise from the trichilemma of the
hair follicle. They should not be mistaken (as they often are) for
sebaceous cysts, which always have a punctum. Pilar cysts have no
punctum and are therefore very mobile underneath the skin.

A less common scalp mass is a *lipoma*. To differentiate it from the pilar cyst, one finds the lipoma to be softer in consistency with a palpable edge and not as freely movable.

A swelling of the scalp of historical interest is called *Pott's puffy tumor*. This is osteomyelitis of the frontal bone from frontal sinusitis resulting in a subperiosteal abscess, causing a soft swelling of the scalp.

Examination of the face from a surgeon's perspective is quite important. Appearance of a patient may give away the diagnosis at the very first sight One example would be *acromegaly*, where prominence of the frontal bones above the eyebrows (often referred to as frontal bossing), protrusion of the jaw, and a thick and enlarged tongue are hallmarks of the disease. Another example would be *Marfan's syndrome*, where a thin, tall body associated with long, thin fingers and toes (arachnodactyly) are highly suggestive of the diagnosis. The former is associated with the pituitary gland and the latter with vascular system abnormalities.

Unilateral or bilateral redness of the face (erythema or cellulitis) can be a sign of a potentially very serious problem. Cellulitis of the face can be a manifestation of *Ludwig's angina* in which the cellulitis is secondary to infection of the floor of the mouth or a tooth abscess. *Ludwig's angina* can be a life-threatening problem causing severe swelling and airway obstruction.

Another type of facial cellulitis that is potentially dangerous is orbital cellulitis. More problematic in children, orbital cellulitis can break the eye socket barrier and cause meningitis. Therefore, it is important to recognize and make the diagnosis early in the course of facial cellulitis so that aggressive treatment can prevent a life-threatening complication. One should be aware of a condition that causes redness of an area of the face with what appears to be a raised rash. This is typical of a streptococcal infection commonly referred to as *erysipelas.*

Some of the obvious facial abnormalities may be diagnostic giveaways. Bulging prominent eyes indicate exophthalmos associated with *thyrotoxicosis.* Increased space between the eyes, known as ocular hypertelorism, is rare and associated with several causes of genetic abnormalities.

A dimple or a sinus tract in front of the tragus of the ear is a developmental abnormality of the first and second branchial arches. The sinus is commonly referred to as a *preauricular sinus.* This should not be mistaken for a punctum of a sebaceous cyst.

Common skin lesions of surgical significance are basal cell and squamous cell carcinomas, of which basal cell carcinoma is more common. The two most common varieties are cystic basal cell carcinoma (BCC) and ulcerating BCC. The cystic BCC is a very subtle finding consisting of a small tiny raised bump with a network of capillaries coursing over it. The ulcerating basal cell carcinoma is usually raised.

Left untreated, the basal cell carcinoma is locally invasive, and its nodular variety on the face or nose might result in a rodent ulcer. Rodent ulcer was thought to result from the bite of a rodent; however it is now known to be untrue.

Oral Cavity

A surgeon's approach to examination of the oral cavity is somewhat different from their medical colleagues. A surgeon's focus is on the floor of the mouth, the tongue, and the tonsillar fossa.

Sometimes it may be necessary to carefully examine the ducts of the major salivary glands.

One should be familiar with rare but interesting physical findings in some children or young adults. These are *ranula* and *lingual thyroid*.

Ranula: Bluish translucent mass located under one or both sides of the tongue in the floor of the mouth. Ranula is named for its resemblance to the ventral aspect of the belly of a frog. (*Rana* in Latin means "frog.") Ranula is a mucocele arising from the sublingual or submaxillary salivary glands or the minor salivary glands of Blandin and Nuhn. Diagnosis and treatment are pretty straight forward.

Lingual thyroid: A mass located on the posterior third of the tongue is an undescended thyroid. It may be the only thyroid tissue in that person. Once the physical exam raises the suspicion of a lingual thyroid, it is imperative to do a thyroid scan, not only to confirm the diagnosis but also to show that there may not be any other thyroid tissue present in the neck.

Any patients with history of smoking, alcohol abuse, and/or betel nut chewing have a higher incidence of carcinoma of the floor of the mouth and tongue. These patients need a very careful inspection and palpation for detecting lesions of the floor of the mouth or the tongue. Early detection is often made by a dentist or an oral surgeon. Any ulcerating lesions should be thought of as malignant in the appropriate age group until proven otherwise.

Carcinoma of the anterior two-thirds of the tongue generally involves the lateral border; however, lesions of the posterior third of the tongue may not be diagnosed until a metastatic lymph node appears in the neck. Sometimes, the workup of a metastatic lymph node in the neck with unknown primary leads to blind biopsies of the posterior third of the tongue with positive results.

Presence of enlarged parotid or submaxillary salivary glands necessitates careful palpation of the ducts of these glands within the oral cavity, as one might find a stone in the duct as a cause for the swelling.

The tonsillar fossa deserves a careful inspection if a patient presents with an enlarged lymph node at the angle of the jaw (jugulodigastric). Usually the tonsillar fossa can be inspected using a tongue depressor; however, use of a laryngeal mirror might give a more complete view of the area.

Parotid Region

The parotid salivary gland extends in front of the ear to past the angle of the jaw into the neck. Parotid gland enlargement, therefore, could involve the entire gland or just the facial or the cervical portion. A mass in front of the tragus of the ear usually represents a mass in the superficial lobe of the parotid gland. A mass just below the angle of the jaw may be in the tail of the parotid gland.

Swelling of the entire parotid gland may be associated with an infectious or an inflammatory process. One of the most common swellings in the parotid region seen in young adults is related to parotitis of mumps. Mumps parotitis involves the entire gland and is quite easily noticeable. This type of parotitis is often bilateral.

Unilateral parotid gland swelling may be a manifestation of an obstructed parotid duct, secondary to a stone in the duct. A careful history is very helpful in making this diagnosis, as the patient would report fluctuations in the size of the swelling with eating as well as associated pain with eating. An examination of the parotid duct inside the oral cavity might reveal a palpable stone in the duct.

An isolated mass at the angle of the jaw located in the tail of the parotid gland is most commonly a Warthin's cyst. It is important to remember that an enlarged lymph node at the angle of the jaw (jugulodigastric) can be easily mistaken for a Warthin's tumor.

A nodule in the superficial lobe of the parotid gland is often a pleomorphic adenoma (also known as mixed tumor). These benign tumors can reach very large sizes if ignored over long periods of time. Bilaterality of a mixed tumor is not uncommon, and therefore, a careful evaluation of the other side is required. If the parotid mass is associated with facial nerve palsy, it is almost always a malignant tumor. Carcinomas of the parotid gland are fortunately rare.

Sometimes lymph node enlargement within the parotid gland may lead to parotid mass. Though rare, one needs to keep in mind that a lymphoma can manifest itself in this way.

NECK

Examination of the neck can be divided into the anterior and the posterior triangles. The anterior triangle includes the submental triangle, the submaxillary triangle, the carotid triangle, and the muscular triangle. The posterior triangle is divided by the inferior belly of the omohyoid muscle into the occipital triangle and the subclavian triangle (also known as supraclavicular triangle).

For ease of description and examination, neck pathology can be described as midline and lateral neck masses.

Midline Neck Masses

1. Submental area mass can be a floor of the mouth lump, showing in the submental area. This would be a *ranula*, which is benign, or a floor-of-the-mouth carcinoma. Enlarged submental lymph nodes also present as upper-neck midline masses. A sublingual salivary gland enlargement may present because of an obstructing stone in its duct, or the salivary gland may be enlarged from a malignant tumor. One should always remember that a submental mass may be something very simple in the subcutaneous tissue such as a lipoma or a sebaceous cyst.

2. Thyroid-region mass in the midline may be a *thyroglossal duct cyst* located either in the suprahyoid region or near the thyroid cartilage. This is generally seen in young adults, and the diagnosis is confirmed by observing movement of the mass upon protrusion of the tongue. Developmentally thyroglossal cysts have a connection to foramen cecum at the base of the tongue, which explains the movement of the cyst with protrusion of the tongue. A more common midline mass in this region would be a thyroid nodule in the isthmus of the thyroid gland. A diagnostic physical finding with any masses connected with thyroid is their movement with the act of swallowing. An uncommon mass in this area would be an enlarged pretracheal lymph node (delphian node). In some cases, an enlarged pyramidal lobe of the thyroid gland might present as a midline neck mass.

3. Suprasternal notch masses are rare. A substernal thyroid mass might present as a mass in the suprasternal notch. If a mass in this area is pulsatile, it is most likely a tortuous

aorta or subclavian artery; however, an aneurysm of the aortic arch may be a rare presentation. A diagnostic sign for an aneurysm of the aortic arch is a tracheal tug. Standing behind the patient, if you hold the _uccessi cartilage up, there is a downward tug with every heartbeat.

Lateral Neck Masses

1. Enlarged submaxillary salivary gland will present as a mass in the submaxillary triangle. A history of fluctuations in the size of the mass, particularly with eating, suggests a benign process likely to be a stone in the submaxillary duct. As indicated earlier, the incidence of malignancy in the submaxillary gland is much higher than the parotid gland. Farther back posterior to this area near the angle of the jaw, a mass is most commonly the jugulodigastric lymph node. Presence of an enlarged node in this area warrants careful evaluation of the tonsillar fossa.

2. Lateral aberrant thyroid is a misnomer given to an enlarged mass in the lateral neck along the carotid artery that represents a metastatic lymph node from papillary carcinoma of the thyroid. It has earned this name because the entire lymph node, often replaced with tumor and histology, might show only the thyroid tissue without any resemblance to a lymph node.

3. *Scrofula* is a name given to tuberculous lymphadenopathy in the neck. This is quite rare, but when it afflicts someone, it presents as a lateral neck mass. Some of the diagnostic features are skin attachment to the underlying mass and, in more advanced cases, presence of sinuses.

4. Branchial cyst, also known as branchial cleft cyst, develops most commonly from an embryological defect of the second branchial cleft. Seen in children or young adults, this lateral neck mass usually presents under the sternocleidomastoid muscle, protruding anteriorly toward the pharynx. These cysts are generally lined with epithelium, which secretes a peculiar fluid. Aspiration of milky fluid from a lateral neck mass is often diagnostic of a branchial cleft cyst.

5. Cystic hygroma is a single or multiloculated cystic structure presenting as a congenital abnormality of the lymphatic system in infancy. This mass presents in the posterior triangle of the neck, and it is commonly located in the supraclavicular area. It is often associated with other chromosomal anomalies, and therefore, genetic testing is important. Fortunately, this is a rare problem.

6. Metastatic lymphadenopathy or lymphoma may present as a lateral neck mass usually along the internal jugular chain of nodes. The metastatic carcinoma lymph nodes tend to be hard in consistency, whereas lymphoma nodes may be rubbery in consistency, particularly if it is a Hodgkin's lymphoma. Metastatic lymph nodes in the neck generally have a primary source in the head and neck area, though in about 15 percent a primary may never be found.

7. Carotid aneurysm and carotid body tumor present as lateral neck masses in the carotid triangle. Both of these are relatively uncommon. Both of these masses may be pulsatile, and sometimes it may be difficult to tell them apart just by clinical exam. Relatively speaking, a carotid body tumor will have transmitted pulsations, as opposed to

33

a carotid aneurysm that will clearly demonstrate expansile pulsations. It was explained earlier how to determine if the pulsations are expansile.

8. Virchow's nodes are a mass of nodes generally in the left supraclavicular area representing metastatic disease from gastric carcinoma. These tend to be on the left side because of the thoracic duct being on the left side.

9. Scalene lymphadenopathy that presents as a mass in the right supraclavicular area may be secondary to metastatic disease from a primary carcinoma of the right lung.

10. Lipomas, sebaceous cysts, and other skin and subcutaneous lesions can be seen in any of the triangles of the neck.

CHEST AND BREAST

CHEST

From a surgical perspective, examination of the chest is just as important as a medical evaluation. The standard methodology of inspection, palpation, percussion, and auscultation applies very well to this area.

Inspection

The most obvious problem might be a deformity of the chest called pectus excavatum. This deformity may vary in severity and can be mild as to give just a sunken appearance of the chest or as severe as to be called a funnel chest. Severe deformity may compromise both respiratory and cardiac function. Presence of this deformity should also alert the examiner that this may be sign of Marfan's syndrome or other associated congenital anomalies.

Look for presence of any scars. A midline sternotomy scar indicates prior open-heart surgery, whereas a scar in the intercostal spaces might be indicative of previous thoracotomy or a MIDCAB (minimally invasive direct coronary artery bypass).

Observe the breathing pattern and notice the respiratory rate. A rapid rate will be quite obvious. Look at the expansion of chest with each inspiration, and note if the right and left sides are symmetrical. Next, look at the accessory muscles of respiration, and see if they are activated. Observe if there is an element of abdominal breathing.

In thin individuals, cardiac pulsations might be visible in the precordium. A strong precordial pulsation visible to the left of the nipple might indicate left ventricular hypertrophy.

Palpation

The first thing to check is to verify symmetrical expansion of both the hemithoraces. This is accomplished by placing the examiner's two hands on the chest wall so that the thumbs are separated from the fingers and the tips of the thumbs meet in the midline over the sternum. Ask the patient to take a deep breath and observe the movement of the thumbs away from the middle as the chest expands. The thumbs should move away from the middle for an equal distance to call the chest expansion symmetrical and equal. If the expansion is asymmetrical, verify the position of the trachea to make sure it is midline.

Feel for any masses or tender spots on the chest wall. A bony mass felt along a rib is most likely a callus from an old rib fracture. Tenderness at the junction of a rib and its cartilage is present in costochondritis.

Feel the apical cardiac pulse in the precordium. If the pulse feels very strong, place the hypothenar eminence on that area to palpate. A strong left ventricular pulse felt with the hypothenar eminence is referred to as a left ventricular heave (indicates left ventricular hypertrophy).

Percussion

Percussion of the chest may have limited value, but it is important for a physician to familiarize himself or herself with its usefulness. The important thing to learn is to recognize the sound and judge the quality of resonance versus dullness. If one sees a patient with a barrel-shaped chest and then on percussion it sounds hyperresonant, the most likely condition is emphysema. A similar hyperresonance associated with shortness of breath and tracheal deviation may be indicative of a pneumothorax. Percussion of the chest in the back with the patient sitting up is helpful in detecting either presence of pleural effusion or consolidation of lobe of the lung.

Percussion of the precordial area can give one an estimate of cardiac size. Percussion is generally started in the left second _ uccession_s space carried downward to the sixth _uccession_s space. The area should extend from the sternum to the midaxillary line.

Auscultation

Auscultation consists of listening to breath sounds and heart sounds, both normal and abnormal. When auscultating the lungs, listen to both the front and the back of the chest. Divide the zones into three, and listen to the apices of the lung, the midlung, and the lung bases. It is also important to listen in the midaxillary area.

Normal Breath Sounds

The normal breath sounds produced by the alveoli of the lungs are called *vesicular* breath sounds. Learn to distinguish these from *bronchial* breath sounds. Bronchial breath sounds are normal when you listen to the tracheo-bronchial tree; however, they are abnormal if you hear them at the lung bases.

Abnormal Breath Sounds

Crackles are moist sounds generally heard at the bases of lungs. Crackles tend to be more pronounced in the inspiratory phase of breathing. The name *crackles* is quite descriptive of what you hear as crackling sounds. These sounds are usually indicative of volume overload in a patient. A typical example would be a patient with congestive heart failure. Sometimes these sounds are also referred to as *rales*.

Wheezes are sounds produced by air trying to squeeze through narrowed breathing passages. These sounds may be low- or high-pitched. Heard best during the expiratory phase of breathing, high-pitched sounds have a whistling quality to them. Wheezes indicate spasm of bronchi or bronchioles. A typical example would be an asthmatic patient with an acute attack.

Stridor is a term referred to noisy breathing, which is sometimes described as a crowing sound. This noisy breathing can be heard without a stethoscope. This is seen more often in patients in acute distress as a result of large airway obstruction and heard best during inspiration.

Friction rub is a grating sound as if two rough surfaces are rubbing against each other. The most common cause would be pleurisy, either secondary to an infectious process or a pulmonary embolus.

Normal Heart Sounds

Auscultation of the heart is done in four areas. For convenience of description, let us number these areas from one to four. Right upper parasternal area between second and third interspace (area 1), left upper parasternal area in the same interspace (area 2), left lower parasternal area from third to the sixth interspace (area 3), and the apex of the heart in the midclavicular line in the fifth and sixth interspace (area 4). Listening to the heart sounds in these four basic areas allows one to evaluate the function of the four heart valves: area 1 for aortic valve function, area 2 for pulmonary valve function, area 3 for tricuspid valve, and area 4 for mitral valve. While listening for heart sounds, one should pay attention to the rate and rhythm of the heart as well.

Abnormal Heart Sounds

Two basic abnormalities are heard. One is a pericardial friction rub, a sound very similar to pleural friction rub but heard synchronous with the heartbeat. The other sound is a murmur. A murmur may be heard during systole or diastole and bears significance in suggesting a diagnosis. Murmurs heard during diastole suggest aortic and pulmonary valve insufficiency and mitral and tricuspid valve stenosis, whereas murmurs heard during systole suggest mitral and tricuspid valve insufficiency and aortic and pulmonary valve stenosis.

Sometimes one hears a murmur in the absence of any pathology. Some call these physiologic murmurs, and these murmurs have little clinical significance. One common example of this is a murmur heard in patients with anemia (sometimes referred to as a hemic murmur).

Heart sounds may be distant for various noncardiac reasons. If the heart sounds are distant, one is first obligated to rule out any cardiac causes for this. The important cardiac causes are pericarditis or pericardial effusion for any reason and vegetations on the valve leaflets softening the heart sounds. Some of the more common noncardiac reasons are COPD with a barrel chest, pneumothorax, morbid obesity, and hypovolemia with hypotension.

BREAST

This is one area of the body where there has been a dramatic change because of promotion of women's health in the recent years. There is increasing acceptance of the fact that there is tremendous value to learning self-examination of the breasts, and more and more women have taken an active role in playing the part. We will first describe a systematic breast exam as a clinician should conduct, and then at the end, there will be a brief note about self-examination. It is generally recommended that a breast examination be conducted in the presence of a chaperone. It is also safer practice not to accept the patient's companion as a chaperone. Breast examination is limited to inspection and palpation. The patient should be asked to bare their upper torso for the examination.

Inspection

Ask the patient to sit up and have her arms by her side. First look for breast symmetry. Some patients may have a natural disparity in the size of the two breasts. If you notice a disparity, ask them if it has always been like that. Sometimes, the size disparity may be related to breast implants or reconstruction. This should be known from taking a detailed history. Look for any indentations, and make sure they are not related to a scar from previous surgery. Remember that the breast tissue extends from the clavicle above to the abdomen below, the sternum medially, and the anterior axillary line laterally, and the so-called tail of breast extends along the pectoral fold to the axilla. Look for any swelling or visible masses in the area of breast tissue as just described. Observe the nipple areola region, and make note of whether the nipple is inverted. If inverted, inquire if this is a recent change. Look for any areolar skin eczema that may be a sign of Paget's disease of the breast. Some patients may present with an area of breast skin that looks like skin of an orange (peau d'orange). This finely dimpled skin appearance is usually a sign of advanced breast cancer and takes that appearance because of plugging of lymphatics of the skin, causing skin edema.

When you see a noticeable swelling of one breast localized to any quadrant, with angry-looking erythematous skin, it can mean one of three things. Firstly, this could be an infection with cellulitis that is seen more commonly in a childbearing age. Secondly, this could be a breast abscess if the swelling is very tender and fluctuant and seen more often in lactating mothers. Thirdly, this can represent an inflammatory carcinoma of the breast that carries a grave prognosis.

The patient is asked to raise her hands above her head, and it should be noted if dimpling or puckering of skin occurs on either side. Again, remember that any scar on the breast from a previous surgical encounter will result in dimpling or puckering of skin upon raising the hands. One is primarily concerned with this finding in the absence of a scar when it is indicative of a possible tumor in the breast with skin attachment.

Next, the patient is asked to place her hands on her waist and brace the shoulders back a bit. This position will make the pectoral muscles taut and push forward any deep-seated mass in the breast to become noticeable. Another maneuver is to have the patient lean forward, thereby allowing the breasts to fall away from the chest

41

wall. This will also cause asymmetry of the breasts if there is skin attachment of a deep-seated mass.

Carefully inspect the axillae to notice any fullness or asymmetry of the axillary fold that might indicate axillary adenopathy.

Palpation

Palpation of the breasts should be done in a systematic fashion. It is best to have the breast divided into six quadrants: the upper outer quadrant, the upper inner quadrant, the lower outer quadrant, the lower inner quadrant, and the subareolar area. The sixth quadrant is the examination of the tail of the breast. Palpation of the breast is conducted both in the sitting-up and lying-down positions. The five-quadrant exam is done with the palmar surface of the fingers held together, and the sixth quadrant is palpated between the fingers posteriorly and the thumb anteriorly.

There are several important considerations while palpating a breast. Examination of a premenopausal patient could be quite different from a postmenopausal patient, and the examination of a premenopausal patient may be different at different phases of her menstrual cycle. This stresses the importance of the history taking to correlate with the findings.

There are premenopausal patients who have either very lumpy breast tissue or extremely dense breast tissue that makes the examination very difficult. These patients fall under the broad category of fibrocystic disease of the breast. Not only is there dense or lumpy breast tissue, but it is also often tender to palpation, particularly during their menstrual period.

Postmenopausal women may have very lumpy breast tissue for a different reason. Their breast tissue undergoes a change from lack of cyclic hormonal influence, and this change is commonly referred to as involution of breast. An involuted breast may present as an alarming lump to a patient who practices self-examination.

When the examining physician finds a mass in the breast by palpation, the first thing to determine is whether it is cystic or solid. It is helpful to note its mobility within the breast tissue and freedom from skin attachment. Document the location accurately by using the face of a clock. For example, a mass in the upper outer quadrant at ten o'clock position gives the next examiner the exact location.

A mass that is freely movable within the breast tissue and is solid by palpation is most commonly a fibroadenoma (often referred to as a breast mouse). A cystic mass in a patient with known history of fibrocystic disease may be aspirated in a clinic setting to confirm the diagnosis.

Presence of a solid breast mass with redness of the overlying skin is highly suspicious of an inflammatory carcinoma of the breast, as mentioned earlier in the inspection of the breast.

Eczema-like lesion of the nipple areola complex should make one examine the subareolar area carefully for presence of a breast mass, the presence of which will suggest a diagnosis of Paget's disease of the nipple. Look for nipple drainage. Sometimes it is necessary to gently squeeze the nipple to demonstrate the drainage. Clear drainage is more common and represents ductal drainage. A milky discharge might indicate presence of a galactocele. Bloody drainage is seen with a ductal papilloma or carcinoma and should always be investigated.

A detailed description of a mass felt in the breast will help arrive at a clinical diagnosis. A mass that is firm to hard in consistency, relatively fixed within the breast tissue, nontender, and having poorly defined borders will be highly suspicious of a breast carcinoma. Skin attachment of this mass with dimpling or puckering would add more credence to the clinical diagnosis of breast cancer.

Once a thorough palpation of the breast is carried out both in the sitting and lying-down positions (lying-down position more suitable for deep palpation of the breast as well as subareolar exam of the breast), attention should be directed toward examination of the lymph node bearing areas.

Though the breast lymphatics drain into internal mammary chain of nodes and supraclavicular chain of nodes, the most pertinent area for clinical exam is the axilla.

The best position to examine the axillary nodes is to have the patient sitting up. Examine patient's left axilla with your right hand and the right axilla with your left hand. Have the patient put her left forearm on your examining right forearm with your hand reaching the axilla. Ask the patient to relax and place your left hand on the patient's left shoulder, depressing it slightly. First feel the lower subpectoral nodes and gain the patient's confidence as you advance your fingertips deep into the axilla. With the patient fully relaxed, and with some gentle pressure on her shoulder, you should be able to reach the apical axillary lymph nodes to evaluate them. Repeat the same procedure for the other axilla, reversing your hands. After examining the axillary nodes, examine the supraclavicular nodes. Obviously, it is not possible to feel the internal mammary chain, and fortunately, it is not involved that often.

Fixation of the breast to the chest wall or feeling enlarged matted lymph nodes in the axilla are generally ominous signs indicating an advanced stage of breast malignancy.

ABDOMINAL EXAMINATION

S urgical students need to learn to examine the abdomen correctly from the very beginning as this would help them for the rest of their medical career. This is also an area of the body where putting the historical facts with the symptomatology and physical findings would help to avoid expensive imaging studies. Examination of the abdomen is complex because it involves examination of not only the viscera and organs within the abdominal cavity, but also the structures located extraperitoneally.

Physical examination of the abdomen is to be carried out in the same systematic fashion, starting with inspection and ending with auscultation. However, this order is changed when one encounters a patient with an acute abdomen. This will be explained in the next chapter.

Inspection

The first thing that is noticeable is the contour of the abdomen and the breathing pattern. Note if the abdomen is distended, flat, or scaphoid (sunken in). Abdominal breathing is seen in patients with COPD. You would also notice shallow breathing in patients who experience pain in the abdomen on breathing normally. Look for any prominent veins coursing over the abdominal wall, which suggest venous collaterals to overcome an obstruction of inferior vena cava. A cluster of very prominent veins around the umbilicus (caput medusae) are seen in patients with advanced cirrhosis of the liver and portal hypertension. It is important to notice any scars on the abdomen or any areas of ecchymosis or discoloration. Bruising around the umbilicus (Cullen's sign) can be seen with intraperitoneal bleeding from any source, though it was described by Cullen for a ruptured ectopic pregnancy. Bruising and ecchymosis in the flanks (Grey Turner's sign) is seen with retroperitoneal processes like hemorrhagic pancreatitis or leaking abdominal aortic aneurysm.

In thin individuals, you might see visible peristalsis in cases of bowel obstruction. Visible peristalsis will also be seen in the absence of bowel obstruction if the patient has a ventral hernia. Abdominal wall defects occur at sites of previous scars when an obvious protrusion is noted in the area. As the fascia is missing from this area, it is not uncommon to see peristalsis in loops of bowel.

If there is protuberance of the abdomen in the midline without the presence of a scar, ask the patient to raise his or her head off the bed. The protuberance becomes very prominent and can be mistaken for a ventral hernia. This is not a hernia but *diastasis recti*. The rectus abdominus muscles from the right and left sides are not together, but separated by a gap, which leads to this phenomenon of diastasis.

In patients with a scaphoid abdomen, an abdominal mass can be visible. A midline abdominal mass that is visibly pulsatile is likely to be an abdominal aortic aneurysm. In similar patients, an enlarged liver and spleen or other abdominal masses might be visible. If you do see an abdominal mass, observe if it has any relationship to respiratory excursions. An enlarged liver or a spleen will move with respirations. If the mass moves directly downward with respirations, it is likely to be liver; however if the mass moves downward and to the right from left, it is likely an enlarged spleen. Obviously, this movement occurs because of the relationship of these organs to the diaphragm.

Abdominal inspection is never complete until both the inguinal areas are looked at. Look at the inguinal areas for any protrusions, visible peristalsis, any skin changes over the protrusions, if any, and any pulsatility to the swellings. A more detailed examination of this area is under the title of "Hernia."

Palpation

The purpose of palpating the abdomen is the following:

1. Feel for any masses
2. Feel for any tenderness
3. Feel for any peritoneal signs

When palpating the abdomen, it is necessary to have the palpating hand at the level of the surface of the abdomen. So it is often essential to raise the bed or the stretcher to gain accurate knowledge with palpating the abdomen. Generally, the tendency is to have the abdominal surface too low for the examination, which results in the examiner unknowingly leaning on the abdomen to produce erroneous results. If, for any reason, it is not possible to raise the patient, the examiner should either sit or kneel to get the examining hand level with the patient's abdomen.

Palpation of the abdomen should be done in a systematic fashion, going quadrant by quadrant. If the patient is presenting with abdominal pain, start the palpation in the opposite quadrant, and get to the symptomatic area last. This helps to build confidence of the patient and avoids any voluntary spasm or guarding of the abdomen. Again, to gain the patient's confidence, first do a superficial palpation of the entire abdomen, and then proceed to do a deep palpation. The superficial palpation is to detect any masses, organomegaly, or any tender spots, and the deeper palpation will give additional information about the same. It has been taught over the years that to avoid voluntary guarding and muscle spasm by the patient, one needs to distract the patient. One of those methods of distraction is to use your stethoscope to pretend to listen but to actually use the diaphragm of the stethoscope to palpate the abdomen for tenderness.

When an abdominal mass is felt, it is important to determine whether this is in the abdominal wall or it is intra-abdominal. With the patient lying down, ask the patient to just raise his or her head off the bed. Any abdominal wall mass that is superficial to the abdominal musculature will become more prominent with this activity. Common examples of these superficial abdominal masses are lipoma, fibrolipoma, fibroma, and neurofibroma. If an abdominal mass becomes less evident and palpable with the raising of head, it is likely an intra-abdominal mass. There are some abdominal wall masses that may not change with this maneuver, the examples of which are a _uccessi tumor or an endometrioma of the abdominal wall. A commonly encountered abdominal wall mass that may be tender to palpation is a hematoma from injections of heparin into the abdominal wall.

If a mass is felt in the upper abdomen, it is important to determine if this is liver or spleen or something else. If you are unable to insinuate your fingers between the mass and the ribcage, it is most likely an enlarged liver. If the mass is in the left upper quadrant, it could be the left lobe of the liver or the spleen, and both of these would not allow insinuation of fingers between the mass and the rib cage. It is relatively easy to make the distinction between the left lobe of the liver and the spleen. Both the spleen and liver move down with inspiration; however, the liver moves straight down, and the spleen moves downward and to the right. Mild to moderate enlargement of the liver is easily palpable, whereas the spleen has to at least double in size before it can become palpable.

A mass palpable in the flank area could be a kidney. A palpable kidney is usually ballotable. Put one hand behind the flank with the palmar surface of the hand facing forward, and put the other hand in front of the flank. As you push with the hand in the back, you will feel the renal mass hit the palpating hand in the front.

A midline nonpulsatile abdominal mass that moves freely in one direction only and not the other can be a mesenteric mass arising from the small bowel mesentery. The mesenteric mass may be a benign cyst or a lymphoma arising from the mesentery.

If any other masses are palpated in the abdomen, it is important to determine if they are tender to palpation. Based on their location, these might be inflammatory masses. If at all possible, evaluate to find out if the abdominal mass is attached to the anterior abdominal wall or if it is fixed to the deeper structures in the abdomen.

A good, detailed palpation of the abdomen can provide a lot of information that may be pertinent to making a physical diagnosis without immediately jumping to imaging modalities.

Percussion

Percussion of the abdomen is helpful for the following:

1. Percuss the outline of a mass or an enlarged organ
2. Percuss for tenderness or presence of peritoneal signs
3. Percuss for presence of free air in the peritoneal cavity (pneumoperitoneum)
4. Percuss for presence of free fluid (ascites)

Percussion is carried out by placing the middle finger of one hand on the abdomen and tapping it with the middle finger of the other hand. Follow the same rules as palpation of the abdomen by starting the examination away from the symptomatic area and coming to the symptomatic area at the end. Percussion of air or a viscous-containing air produces a resonant sound as opposed to an organ or a solid mass that produces a dull sound. Presence of fluid will also produce a dull sound. By percussing from the umbilicus up toward left or right upper quadrants, resonance will change to dullness as one approaches the liver and spleen. If the dullness is appreciated well below the rib cage, it would generally mean either an enlarged liver or spleen (more common) or a relatively uncommon condition of ptosis of the organs when the organs drop down.

Absence of liver dullness is a classic sign of pneumoperitoneum (free air in the abdominal cavity). As free air in the abdomen tends to rise to an under-the-diaphragm position, percussion resonance continues over the liver area to the lung. The most common cause of pneumoperitoneum is post-op open abdominal operation. The second most common cause is a perforated viscus (perforated peptic ulcer is on the top of the list).

Percussion is a very sensitive test for evaluating peritoneal irritation from an inflammatory process. For example, in cases of acute appendicitis, there will be significant tenderness to percussion over the McBurney's point (described in the next chapter).

When a patient presents with ascites, it is possible to make this diagnosis by percussion. In the presence of free fluid in the abdominal cavity, the air containing bowel tends to float on top of the fluid. So if you percuss the front of the abdomen with the patient lying flat, there will be resonance in the middle of the abdomen and dullness as you move away from the middle. The next step is to ask the patient to turn slightly to one side or the other with which the floating bowel will again move to the top of the fluid, and the area of dullness to percussion will shift. This is the classic "shifting-dullness sign," indicating presence of ascites. The shifting dullness may be difficult to demonstrate if the amount of fluid in the abdomen is limited. In these circumstances, the patient is asked to assume a knee-chest posture, and percussion around the umbilicus in that posture would reveal dullness as the fluid tends to gravitate to the most dependent position. It has been estimated that as little as 150 ml of fluid may be detectable when examined in a knee-chest position.

Some rare post-operative complications may be diagnosed with careful percussion; for example, a large area of resonance in the left upper quadrant post-op with upper abdominal distress may be seen in acute gastric dilatation. Similarly, a massive dilatation of cecum with threatening perforation could be percussed and suspicion raised clinically.

Auscultation

Auscultation of the abdomen establishes the following:

1. Presence or absence of bowel sounds
2. Presence of any abnormal intestinal sounds
3. Presence or absence of bruits

The frequency of bowel sounds is variable. There may be as few as one or two sounds per minute or as many as twenty to thirty per minute. Under normal circumstances, bowel sounds are fewer (hypoactive) during sleep and very frequent (hyperactive) after eating. One should really listen to the abdomen for a minute or two before declaring it to be a silent abdomen. A silent abdomen indicates one of two things: either the bowel sounds are absent because of ileus (also referred to as paralytic ileus) or the bowel activity (peristalsis) has ceased because of severe peritoneal infectious process. These two things may also require very different approaches to treatment. A silent abdomen because of ileus is generally managed with conservative treatment, whereas a silent abdomen as part of an acute abdominal catastrophe would require emergent surgical intervention.

There are basically two types of abnormal sounds one can detect while listening with a stethoscope. Bowel sounds that are so loud that you can hear them even without a stethoscope but then are confirmed with the stethoscope (borborygmi) are associated with intestinal obstruction. These sounds are heard intermittently with the waves of peristalsis and are often associated with colicky abdominal pain. These loud sounds need distinction from loud peristalsis or growling sounds often heard after eating or even when one is hungry. These normal loud sounds are painless.

Another abnormal sound heard occasionally is referred to as _uccession splash. This is a sloshing sound heard best in the left upper quadrant with a stethoscope upon shaking the patient, indicating presence of a large amount of air and fluid in the stomach. Succussion splash is most commonly present in patients with gastric outlet obstruction.

Auscultation can detect presence of an abdominal bruit (a whooshing sound produced due to turbulent blood flow through a narrowed artery. Abdominal bruit is not an uncommon finding in older individuals. With some practice and experience, an examiner can learn to distinguish a bruit heard because of aortic disease from bruits heard as a result of the narrowing of the large visceral branches of the aorta. As a general rule, bruits heard in the midline may represent narrowing of the celiac or superior mesenteric artery. Bruits heard in the midabdomen going toward the flank are likely to be from the renal arteries, and bruits over the lower quadrants of the abdomen are from the iliac arteries. Obviously, correlation with the presenting symptoms is always helpful in arriving at a diagnosis.

ACUTE ABDOMEN

An acute abdomen may be defined as an abdominal catastrophe of abrupt onset that, if undiagnosed and untreated, may be fatal. The stress here should be on diagnosis because a number of acute abdominal catastrophes are treatable with early intervention, and most often, that intervention is surgical. Therefore, it is incumbent upon every student of surgery to be able to diagnose an acute abdomen. Some only refer to an acute abdomen as an acute abdominal process causing peritonitis; however, this limited view would exclude some life-threatening acute abdominal events, like a ruptured abdominal aortic aneurysm.

Accurate history and the sequence of events combined with the physical findings are very important in arriving at the diagnosis. The most common symptoms of severe abdominal pain of sudden onset, nausea, vomiting, fever, and syncope episode may be accompanied with a variety of other symptoms.

HISTORY

Presentation with abdominal pain, nausea, and vomiting is quite common. It is of utmost importance to know the sequence of these symptoms. The etiology of abdominal pain following nausea and vomiting will be very different from nausea and vomiting following the abdominal pain. Always keep in mind the nonsurgical causes of an acute abdomen, and in a female patient, it is essential to know the menstrual and gynecologic history.

Pain

Pain is probably the most important of all the other symptoms of an acute abdomen. Note the following:

a. *Onset of pain and duration:* Was the pain of sudden onset? Or was it of gradual onset, building up in intensity? If the onset of pain followed ingestion of a fatty meal, it is likely to be an acute biliary colic. Severe abdominal pain following a bout of retching and vomiting may be a tear at the gastroesophageal junction (Mallory-Weiss) or a perforated esophagus (Boerhaave's). The duration of symptoms have a bearing on the type of surgical treatment offered.

b. *Location:* Location of pain itself might give one a clue about the underlying pathology. For example, epigastric pain may be associated with a perforated peptic ulcer or pancreatitis. Right upper-quadrant pain may be from gall bladder or biliary pathology; left upper-quadrant pain may be related to gastroesophageal or splenic pathology. Midabdominal or periumbilical pain is often associated with acute appendicitis or small bowel obstruction. Right lower-quadrant pain is associated with acute appendicitis or female adnexal problems, and left lower quadrant pain is often due to acute diverticulitis. Flank pain radiating to the

55

lower quadrants is seen with ureteral colic. Lower abdominal pain in a female patient should always make you think of ob-gyn pathology like ovulation pain, ectopic pregnancy, or problems associated with the uterus, tubes, and ovaries. All this information pertaining to the location of pain is a general guideline, and it is not unusual to see some cross over. The diagnoses mentioned here are the more common conditions and by no means cover the entire list of possibilities.

c. *Character*: The character of pain may vary from a dull ache to sharp, stabbing pain. The pain may be continuous or intermittent. If continuous sharp, stabbing pain is suddenly ameliorated without doing anything, it may be an ominous sign representing perforation of a viscus. Sharp pain that is intermittent and that comes and goes may be associated with peristalsis and is often indicative of intestinal obstruction. Constant dull pain may be seen with ischemic bowel or an inflammatory process in the abdomen.

d. *Factors influencing pain*: It is helpful to know what makes the pain better or worse. For example, if the patient volunteers the information that on his/her car ride to the hospital, every bump in the road was very painful, this would be highly suspicious of peritonitis. If severe epigastric pain was better with the patient sitting up in bed and leaning forward, it would point toward pancreatitis as a likely diagnosis. If a patient tells you that the right lower-quadrant pain was somewhat relieved by keeping the right leg flexed and drawn up, then the patient might be giving you a diagnosis of acute appendicitis. If you find a patient writhing in pain and it appears that no position or maneuver seems to relieve it, then think of renal colic from a ureteral stone.

When a patient presents with an acute abdomen with suspicion of acute appendicitis or bowel obstruction and claims that their severe pain has suddenly subsided without pain medication, it would often indicate perforation of the appendix or bowel perforation. Relief of severe colicky pain after a bout of vomiting would be highly suggestive of acute intestinal obstruction.

Nausea and Vomiting

As mentioned earlier, the sequence of the onset of these symptoms is important. Nausea and vomiting may not always represent bowel obstruction, though this will be the leading component of the symptom complex of any bowel obstruction. Nausea is a very nonspecific symptom and is often associated with the severity of pain. A detailed description of the vomiting is very helpful in prioritizing the differential diagnosis.

1. *Onset*: Nausea and vomiting starting immediately after eating is likely to be food poisoning or gastroenteritis. The timing of onset of vomiting is often related to where the obstruction is in the gastrointestinal tract. Obviously, early onset after ingestion of food will be from gastric-outlet obstruction, whereas large intestinal obstruction will manifest vomiting much later. Always inquire about what was ingested prior to the onset of symptoms. Overuse of NSAIDs can lead to an acute ulcer with perforation of the stomach. Some patients

experience nausea and vomiting just from the severity of pain without any underlying obstruction.

2. *Character*: It is pertinent to know the details of the character of the vomiting. The different types of vomitus may be blood, bilious material, nonbilious material, or feculent material. Vomiting of blood is seen in bleeding peptic ulcer, bleeding gastroesophageal varices, or an aortoduodenal fistula. All these emergent problems have serious consequences and need early and accurate diagnosis. Vomiting of undigested food is seen in patients with gastric outlet obstruction. Bilious vomiting suggests proximal small-intestinal obstruction, and feculent vomiting indicates distal small bowel or large-intestinal obstruction.

3. *Associated symptoms*: Nausea and vomiting associated with diarrhea is a hallmark of gastroenteritis. Severe retching and vomiting followed by acute abdominal pain and or upper-GI hemorrhage should make one think of a Mallory-Weiss tear at the GE junction or an esophageal perforation (Boerhaave's syndrome).

Fever

When patients with acute abdominal symptoms present with fever, it lends more credence to the diagnosis of an acute abdomen. Generally a symptom of an inflammatory process in the body, fever might indicate the severity of the problem. Low-grade fever is nonspecific; however, any fever over 101 degrees Fahrenheit should be paid attention to. Patients presenting with high fevers associated with abdominal symptoms may have a free or a contained perforation of a viscus with peritonitis. Fever may also be a marker of progression of a nonstrangulating bowel obstruction to strangulation or progression of ischemic bowel to frank gangrene.

Always remember that children behave very differently from adults. Children tend to have a much higher febrile response than adults, and a febrile convulsion might be very alarming to the examiner.

In addition to history of the symptoms outlined above, it is important to obtain history of the following:

1. Is the patient sexually active?
2. Has the patient recently travelled abroad?
3. Is there a family history of such problems?
4. Has the patient ever experienced such symptoms before?

PHYSICAL EXAMINATION

Starting with the appearance of the patient, the standard protocol of inspection, palpation, percussion, and auscultation of the abdomen is carried out. The only change in examination of a patient with acute abdomen is that auscultation should precede palpation and percussion. This change in sequence is to avoid a false impression of hearing bowel sounds in an otherwise silent abdomen as palpation might cause some peristaltic activity.

Inspection

Observe what the patient is doing. A restless patient is often in pain and cannot find a comfortable position. This is usually seen in patients with ureteral colic, pancreatitis, or a major abdominal catastrophe. A patient lying with the knees bent or curled up on the side is generally indicative of peritonitis. Flexing the hips and bending the knees tilts the pelvis and relaxes the anterior abdominal muscles, thus giving relief of pain in cases of peritonitis.

A patient sitting up in bed and leaning forward to get relief from pain is typically seen in pancreatitis. It is essential to have the patient's abdomen exposed during examination. Note the breathing pattern. If the patient's breathing is shallow, it may be because breathing normally causes more pain, and this will point toward pathology in the upper abdomen. Look for presence of any scars on the abdomen. Carefully observe the groin areas for any hernia bulges. Visible peristalsis might be seen in thin patients with bowel obstruction. This will not be seen if there is distention of the abdomen. If there are hernia bulges in the groin area, look for any visible peristalsis in the bulge, and pay attention to the overlying skin. Redness or edema of skin overlying a hernia bulge has serious consequences as this usually indicates compromised bowel underneath.

Auscultation

Remember to warm up your stethoscope with your hands before placing it on the patient. Listen in all four quadrants of the abdomen, and listen for several minutes before declaring it to be a silent abdomen. It is a good practice to start listening in a quadrant away from where the symptoms are. This gains the patient's confidence and facilitates the palpation and percussion to follow. Acute nonstrangulating intestinal obstruction will present with high-pitched bowel sounds, which are intermittent and coincide with peristaltic activity. If bowel sounds are audible over hernia bulges, it indicates presence of bowel in the hernia sac.

A patient with significant abdominal pain is afraid that the examiner's hand is likely to push the abdomen and cause a lot of pain. This fear results in the patient voluntarily guarding the abdomen so the examination becomes difficult. One method to overcome the patient's fear has been taught for decades by experienced clinicians. This method is to use the stethoscope for palpating the abdomen. As the patient thinks that you are listening to the abdomen, a gentle palpation can be carried out using the diaphragm of the stethoscope while the patient remains distracted. This method of examination is particularly effective in patients with peritonitis.

In an acute abdomen, auscultation of the abdomen has limited usefulness as indicated above. In majority of cases, it is used mainly to establish presence or absence of bowel sounds and the character of the bowel sounds.

Palpation

Palpation is considered a more important part of the abdominal examination for an acute abdomen. Applying the correct methodology for palpating the abdomen is crucial. Some of this was mentioned earlier under the general principles of physical examination. The palpating hand should be flat with the surface of the abdomen. This could mean either raising the bed of the patient or lowering yourself by sitting or kneeling by the bedside. If this point is ignored, the palpation ends up being heavy-handed and may elicit more pain and tenderness than actually present. It cannot be repeated enough to remind oneself to start palpating farthest away from where the symptoms are. A gentle superficial palpation of all quadrants is done to evaluate for signs of peritoneal irritation (peritonitis).

In patients with acute abdominal pain where appendicitis is suspected, ask the patient if they can point with one finger where the pain is. If the patient puts a finger directly on the McBurney's point (a spot a third of the way from the anterior superior iliac spine on the right and the umbilicus), it is highly suggestive of acute appendicitis. Palpation at this point will elicit pain and tenderness. Another sign of acute appendicitis is to develop hypersensitivity of skin in the Sherren's triangle. This is a triangle in the right lower quadrant, bounded by the anterior superior iliac spine, umbilicus, and pubic tubercle. Just gently stroking the skin in this area is uncomfortable. Palpating the left lower quadrant and suddenly releasing the abdominal wall causes pain in the right lower quadrant (Rovsing's sign). This is another positive sign for acute appendicitis. There are other causes of an acute abdomen with pain in the right lower quadrant, which need consideration in the differential diagnosis of acute appendicitis. In a female patient of childbearing age, an ectopic pregnancy, a ruptured or torsed ovarian cyst, a tubo-ovarian abscess, a torsion of a fibroid uterus, and a red degeneration of fibroid during pregnancy can all mimic acute appendicitis. A ureteral colic is always in the differential diagnosis of acute appendicitis; however, it is accompanied by appropriate flank tenderness and blood in the urine. One of the uncommon reasons for severe right lower-quadrant pain with unusually high fever and right lower-quadrant tenderness may be from acute prostatitis. This diagnosis can be easily established by a rectal exam and palpation of the prostate and examination of any discharge from the penis.

Palpating the right upper quadrant deeply and asking the patient to take a deep breath might result in the patient suddenly ceasing respiration because of severe pain (Murphy's sign). This finding is suggestive of acute cholecystitis. A palpable tender mass in the right upper quadrant may be a hydrops of the gall bladder, where an obstructing stone in the cystic duct causes painful distention of the gall bladder, making it palpable. The gall bladder mass can be distinguished from a liver mass by the fact that the examining hand can insinuate the fingers between the mass and the rib cage. One is unable to do that with a liver mass.

Tenderness to palpation in the epigastric area is suggestive of pancreatitis. One needs to tie in the history and symptoms with the findings on examination to come up with a diagnosis. A patient who presents with an acute abdomen and has a history of alcohol abuse or biliary tract disease and has tenderness to deep palpation in the epigastrium is most likely to have acute pancreatitis.

When a patient presents with left lower-quadrant pain of acute onset and has significant tenderness to palpation in the left lower quadrant with evidence of peritoneal irritation (rebound tenderness), the most likely diagnosis is acute diverticulitis. If this happens to be a female in the childbearing age, an ectopic pregnancy or a tubo-ovarian abscess or a ruptured ovarian cyst should be in the differential diagnosis.

Any patient presenting with a history of syncope, severe back pain, and a palpable abdominal mass is likely experiencing a leaking abdominal aortic aneurysm and needs immediate attention.

Acute abdominal pain associated with a tender mass in the groin is suspicious of an incarcerated hernia with possible bowel obstruction. Under these circumstances, carefully examine the groin area with the mass. If there are changes in the overlying skin in the form of erythema, edema, and severe tenderness to palpation, it is likely that the patient has a strangulated hernia (has compromised circulation to the loop of bowel in the hernia sac).

Percussion

Percussion is a very useful physical diagnostic tool in evaluating a patient with an acute abdomen. Placing the middle finger of one hand flat on the surface of the abdomen and tapping with the middle finger of the other hand is a very important part of the examination. First of all, percussion is a very sensitive method of detecting peritoneal signs (indicating peritonitis). Proceed in a systematic fashion just like palpation starting to percuss in the quadrant of the abdomen farthest away from the symptomatic area. Again, this is to gain the patient's confidence, allowing the patient to be relaxed. You can get a lot more accurate information when the patient is relaxed than when the patient tenses up and starts voluntarily guarding the abdomen for fear of pain.

Percussing over the liver in the right upper quadrant and demonstrating absence of liver dullness is a reliable sign of presence of free air in the abdomen (indicating a perforated viscus).

It is possible to percuss the outline of a large stomach in the left upper quadrant as in acute gastric dilatation.

Point tenderness to percussion over the McBurney's point is suggestive of acute appendicitis. Percussion over a groin mass might tell you that it is an air-filled loop of bowel in the hernia.

Summary

It is helpful to summarize the differential diagnosis of various acute abdominal events based on location of pain, associated symptoms, and physical findings in men and women.

Differential Diagnosis of Acute Appendicitis

Right lower-lobe pneumonia, acute cholecystitis, acute pancreatitis, perforated peptic ulcer, Crohn's ileitis, mesenteric adenitis, ureteral colic, acute prostatitis, right testicular torsion, acute diverticulitis, and additional diagnosis to consider in women, mittelschmerz, ectopic pregnancy, PID, torsion or rupture of ovarian cyst, endometriosis, and red degeneration in a fibroid.

The list of differential diagnosis cannot be complete unless we included some rare conditions like a rectus sheath hematoma, acute porphyria, abdominal crisis of tabes dorsalis, and diabetic ketoacidosis (DKA).

Differential Diagnosis of Perforated Peptic Ulcer

Myocardial infarction, acute gastritis, perforated esophagus (Boerhaave's syndrome), acute pancreatitis, acute cholecystitis, acute chledocholithiasis, acute cholangitis, and rarely, aortic dissection.

HERNIA

Hernia may be defined as protrusion of a viscus or part of a viscus through a normal or abnormal opening in the abdomen. Hernias may be external or internal, the external being a lot more common than the internal. The most common location for external hernias is the groin. A groin hernia may be inguinal or femoral. The inguinal hernia is the most common hernia in both males and females; however, the femoral hernia is much more common in the females; as the femoral hernias come through the femoral ring into the femoral triangle, a larger pelvis makes these hernias more common in the female gender.

The inguinal hernias may be of indirect or direct variety. The inguinal hernia is indirect when it comes through the internal abdominal ring into the inguinal canal, whereas the direct hernia results from a deficient posterior wall of the inguinal canal.

A physical exam is never complete unless one has stripped the patient to below the groin level and checked for hernias. Following the pattern in this book, we will conduct the physical exam in the same order of inspection, palpation, percussion, and auscultation.

Inspection

Look for presence of a bulge in the groin area. Sometimes it is obvious if the bulge is above the inguinal ligament or below the ligament. Obviously, the bulge above the ligament is an inguinal hernia, and the bulge below is likely a femoral hernia. The bulge in the case of a femoral hernia will be more medial, closer to the pubis than an inguinal hernia. Remember that sometimes a femoral hernia will come through the femoral canal, and as it gets larger, it may take a route cephalad and present as an inguinal mass. It is advisable to examine the patient in both a standing and a recumbent position. If there is a noticeable bulge on standing that disappears on lying down, this would suggest a direct inguinal hernia. The patient might give a history of having noticed or felt a bulge, but none is present at the time of examination. Ask the patient to cough and observe if a bulge appears on coughing. In a male, note if the swelling extends into the scrotum, which makes it an inguinoscrotal hernia. These inguinoscrotal hernias are indirect hernias. If one notices a scrotal swelling, it is important to distinguish a scrotal hernia from a hydrocele of the tunica vaginalis. It is not possible to make that distinction by inspection alone.

Inspection of the inguinal hernia includes evaluating the skin overlying the bulge. Look for skin changes in the form of erythema or edema. If these skin changes are present with a painful bulge in the groin, there should be high suspicion for strangulating hernia.

Carefully observe if there is any visible peristalsis in the groin mass, which would automatically indicate presence of bowel in the hernia sac. If there is visible peristalsis, watch for patient's facial expression when you observe the peristalsis. A correlation of grimacing with the visible peristalsis would make one suspicious of bowel obstruction within the hernia.

Examination for hernias in an infant can be quite challenging. Often the mother would report having seen a bulge when the infant cried and it disappeared at other times. One should know that in infants, the hernias are a result of the processus vaginalis remaining patent, and therefore, the male infants would have a combination of hernia hydrocele. If the child does not cry during your examination, you may have to make the diagnosis by palpation.

Palpation

The most important part of the physical examination of an inguinal or femoral hernia is palpation. In a female patient, palpate the inguinal canal with the hand and ask the patient to cough. One would feel an impulse on coughing even if there is no obvious bulge. In a male patient, invaginate the scrotum with your index finger into the inguinal canal, and ask the patient to cough. If the impulse on coughing is felt by the tip of the index finger, it is most likely an indirect inguinal hernia. If the impulse on coughing is felt by the pulp of the index finger, it is likely a direct inguinal hernia.

When patients present with an obvious bulge, one attempts to see if this can be reduced. An easily reducible hernia makes it a nonemergent or nonurgent situation.

Tenderness to palpation or pain in attempting to reduce the hernia should raise a red flag. This situation may have to be attended to urgently. It is important to learn the correct technique for reducing a hernia. Most nonreducible (incarcerated) hernias are indirect inguinal hernias or femoral hernias. Place the index finger and thumb on either side of the opening where the hernia is likely coming from, then gently squeeze the hernia with the other hand, directing it with your finger and thumb to guide it back. Never use excessive pressure or force, for fear of causing the hernia with compromised contents to get reduced into the abdomen with the sac containing them. This is called reduction en masse, with a potential danger of pushing dead bowel into the abdomen with dire consequences.

When the scrotal hernia and hydrocele get very large in a male patient, it is difficult to tell them apart. There are several features on palpation that help make the diagnosis of one versus the other. In an inguinoscrotal hernia, it is not possible to get above the scrotal swelling. If the swelling is reducible, it is obviously a hernia, but even if the swelling is nonreducible, you can always palpate the testicle at the bottom of the swelling. It is possible to get above the scrotal swelling if it is a hydrocele, but impossible to feel the testicle as the fluid accumulation is between the layers of tunica vaginalis and tunica albuginea. A hydrocele can be transilluminated, and one would see the shadow of a testicle in the transillumination.

On examination of a male infant who does not cooperate by crying during the exam, palpation of the root of the scrotum will help make the diagnosis. Feeling the root of the scrotum of an infant with a hernia hydrocele combination (often seen together) by grasping between the index finger and thumb gives one the feeling of a silk glove. Therefore, this has been described as a silk-glove sign, and depending on how convinced the examiner is, it is graded from 1+ to 4+ silk-glove sign.

Percussion and Auscultation

Percussion and auscultation add little to the physical examination; however, they should not be neglected. Percussion over the hernia may elicit pain, which indicates that urgent attention is needed. Percussion may also reveal tympany over the hernia, indicating presence of bowel as a content of the hernia. Percussion of the rest of the abdomen, revealing significant tympany, makes one suspicious of obstructed bowel with distention, possibly from an incarcerated hernia. Percussion of the abdomen may also elicit tenderness, which makes one suspicious of peritoneal signs (peritonitis).

Auscultation over the hernia might reveal bowel sounds, thereby confirming presence of bowel in the hernia. Presence of bowel sounds assures the examiner of the viability of the bowel. It is beneficial to auscultate the abdomen again to make sure that it is not a silent abdomen.

Review of Types of Hernias

Broad classification of hernias is into direct and indirect. The most common structure involved in a direct hernia is the urinary bladder.

The following are different types of indirect hernias:

1. Sliding hernia: An organ or viscus forms part of the wall of the hernia sac.
2. Richter's hernia: Part of the circumference of the bowel is trapped in a hernia.
3. Littre's hernia: When the content of the hernia sac is a Meckel's diverticulum
4. Pantaloon hernia: When there is both direct and indirect hernia sacs like a pair of pants
5. Amyand's hernia: When appendix is in the hernia
6. Busse's hernia: When there is a testicle in the hernia

Points to Remember

1. The most common groin hernia is an inguinal hernia, though a femoral hernia is more common in a female.

2. The most common sliding hernia is a hiatus hernia.

3. Any organ or viscus that is totally intraperitoneal cannot be a part of a sliding hernia. There are only two structures that fit this description, namely the small intestine and ovary.

4. Physical examination of the abdomen is never complete unless the groins are checked for hernias.

5. Signs and symptoms to look for when an incarcerated hernia becomes strangulated hernia are constant pain at the site, redness and edema of the overlying skin, fever, tachycardia, and a rising WBC count.

71

EXTERNAL GENITALIA, RECTAL, AND PELVIC EXAMINATION

EXTERNAL GENITALIA

There is a lot more to examination of external genitalia in a male as opposed to a female. The female examination is limited to the labia majora, the vaginal introitus, and the urethral meatus. The external genitalia in a female are also referred to as vulva. Vulvar neoplasm is generally vulvar carcinoma. In postmenopausal women, there should be a high index of suspicion for any vulvar lesions.

Inspection of the vulva might also reveal cysts of the Bartholin's glands. Bartholin's glands (one each) are located on either side of the introitus. There may be varicose veins of the labia majora noticed more often during pregnancy; however, residual varicosities may be seen even in a nonpregnant state.

A lesion of the urethral orifice is noted in some patients. This is a raw-appearing raised lesion of the posterior lip of the urethra, which is called a *urethral caruncle*. These can be painful lesions and are chronically infected.

Examination of external genitalia in a male patient involves examination of the penis and the scrotum. One of the relatively common conditions involving the penis is *phimosis*, which is inability to retract the foreskin over the glans of the penis. An opposite of this condition which is much less common is *paraphimosis*, where the foreskin remain retracted proximal to the head of the penis and it is not possible to bring it down over the glans penis. If this condition is persistent, it can compromise the blood flow to the head of the penis, resulting in gangrene in the most severe cases.

Look for any congenital abnormalities like *hypospadias* when a lot of patients may be unaware of their own abnormality. Feel the shaft of the penis for any abnormal thickening or curvature indicating *Peyronie's disease*, which may affect as high as 10 percent of the males.

Ulcers on the penis are more commonly seen in venereal disease; however, it is important to remember to carefully inspect the glans for presence of malignant ulcers (squamous cell carcinoma).

On examination of the scrotum, the very first observation should be to make sure both testicles are present. Absence of a testicle means either it has not descended or it was surgically removed. In an undescended testicle, it is important to determine if it is located in the groin or has remained intra-abdominal.

Palpation of the testicle will determine if there is any tenderness as seen in orchitis. At the upper pole of the testicle, it is possible to appreciate the epididymis. Feel for any abnormality or tenderness of the epididymis. In some instances, a cyst of the epididymis can be detected just by careful palpation. Tenderness of the epididymis is associated with epididymitis or epididymo-orchitis. A swollen testicle can be appreciated by palpation as there is the other side

73

to compare. A painless testicular mass is a testicular tumor until proven otherwise.

A scrotal swelling is usually a benign process. The most common cause of scrotal swelling is a scrotal hernia. It is an inguinoscrotal hernia, and as described before, on examination, you are unable to get above the swelling. You should be able to feel the testicle at the bottom of the swelling, and the swelling may also be reducible. If the scrotal swelling is such that you can get above the swelling and you are unable to feel the testicle, it is likely a *hydrocele* of the *tunica vaginalis*. This swelling should transilluminate nicely, which will then be diagnostic.

How do you distinguish a *hydrocele* from a *hematocele*? This is done by three features. Firstly, the *hematocele* is firm to hard to palpation as opposed to fluctuant. Secondly, a *hematocele* will not transilluminate, and thirdly, when you weigh the scrotum in the palm of your hand, the *hematocele* feels much heavier than a *hydrocele*.

RECTAL EXAMINATION

Physical examination of a patient is incomplete without a rectal exam. The information obtained by a rectal exam that is independent of gender includes the evaluation of the rectum and anal canal. The patient is placed in a left lateral position appropriately draped to protect their modesty. The patient is asked to take a nice, deep breath and relax, and warn the patient before you insert your well-lubricated finger into the anal canal and rectum. Examination is conducted with an index finger, the average length of which is about seven centimeters. As you traverse the anal canal, appreciate the tone of the anal sphincter, and upon entering the rectum, note the presence of stool in the rectal vault. If stool is present, note the consistency of the stool. Carefully palpate for any masses, polyps, or malignant tumors.

Normally, internal hemorrhoids cannot be palpated unless they are prolapsing out of the anal canal or have thrombosis. A painful rectal exam is indicative of a fissure in ano, and if present, do a careful exam of the area. An acute fissure in ano is accompanied by spasm of the anal sphincter, which is the primary reason for the pain. A chronic fissure tends to be less painful and will usually show some fibrotic changes in its bed. Often the fissure is posterior and is generally accompanied by an overhanging tag of skin referred to as a sentinel pile.

In a male patient, turn the pulp of your finger anteriorly, and palpate the prostate gland. Feel the prostate for any enlargement or hardness in consistency. Tenderness and a boggy feel to the prostate are seen in cases of prostatitis. Faced with suspicion of prostatitis, do a gentle massage of the prostate to obtain urethral discharge for gram stain and culture.

Sometimes you will find multiple openings in the perineum discharging urine. These are the result of stricture of urethra causing recurrent periurethral abscesses that eventually end up as multiple urinary fistulae. This condition is often referred to as a watering-can perineum.

In a female patient, particularly a virgin with an intact hymen, rectal examination can be used to examine the pelvic organs.

Look for openings in the perianal area discharging purulent material or feces. These are fistulae in ano. If the opening is anterior to the anal canal, these fistulae tend to have a straight course opening into the rectum. If the opening is posterior to the anal canal, the fistulous tract follows a curved course before opening into the rectum (Goodsall's rule).

At the conclusion of the digital examination, one usually finds some stool at the very tip of the finger. It should be routine to perform a guaiac test to look for presence of occult blood.

PELVIC EXAMINATION

A lot of information can be gained by a well-conducted pelvic exam. Unfortunately, these days we are too quick to get a pelvic ultrasound rather than do a thorough pelvic examination. A male physician conducting a pelvic exam should always have a chaperone. From a medical-legal standpoint, it is advisable not have a patient's family member be the chaperone. The patient's modesty needs to be respected, and the patient should be appropriately covered while the pelvic exam is being done.

As we have done before, we start with inspection before we palpate, which means we do a vaginal speculum examination before a digital exam. Select an appropriate-sized vaginal speculum, and with the patient in a lithotomy position, inspect the vagina and cervix. It is important to have a good light source to be able to inspect properly. Look for any vaginal abnormalities like a rectovaginal fistula. Look carefully at the cervix for any abnormality suspicious of neoplasia. This is a good time to do a pap smear. At the conclusion of the speculum exam, proceed with digital examination

The examination consists of first doing a vaginal exam, followed by a bimanual pelvic exam. The vaginal exam is done with two fingers (index and middle), well lubricated, always communicating with the patient as to what is being done. Feel for any abnormalities of the vagina itself, and then proceed to examine the uterus. By examining the cervix and the fundus of the uterus, the position of the uterus is noted first. When a uterus is tipped forward, the cervix will point backward, and this is called an anteverted uterus. The reverse of this with the uterus tipped back and the cervix forward is a retroverted uterus. An anteverted uterus is more common than a retroverted uterus. When the uterus is tipped back without the cervix changing its position, it is referred to as a retroflexed uterus. Sometimes, a retroverted or retroflexed uterus is associated with back pain or dysmenorrhea. The cervix can be moved or wiggled to see if it elicits any pain. Painful movement of the cervix is often associated with pelvic inflammatory disease (PID).

Examine on either side of cervix, the spaces called fornices, to feel the adnexa. Any abnormality of the fallopian tube (e.g., hydrosalpinx) or the ovary (a cyst or neoplasm) can be appreciated in the fornix. After doing this, the next step would be a bimanual exam.

In a bimanual pelvic exam, fingers of one hand are in the vagina, and the fingers of other hand are placed suprapubically to palpate both the uterus and the ovaries. The uterus is palpated with the other hand in the midline above the pubis, whereas the ovaries are palpated with the other hand in the lower quadrant of the abdomen. You can not only feel the pelvic organs, but also have a pretty good idea about the size of these organs to appreciate normalcy or enlargement. A tender adnexal mass by bimanual exam usually suggests a tubo-ovarian abscess.

A bimanual pelvic exam in thinner individuals will allow you to detect fibroids uteri, ovarian cysts or neoplasia, and/or other pelvic pathology.

VASCULAR EXAMINATION

V ascular system is a system of the body, which can be evaluated fairly accurately by a good, thorough physical examination at the bedside. Examination of the vascular system is unique in that it spans the entire body from head to toes. One of the exceptions to our usual method of examination of various parts of the body is that percussion has no value in evaluating the vascular system except for eliciting Tinel's sign.

It is more convenient to divide the vascular system into the arterial system and venous system for evaluation as they are quite different.

ARTERIAL SYSTEM

Inspection

The appearance of the patient (usually a male patient) can sometimes shed light on possible vascular problems they might have. A good example of this is a patient with Marfan's syndrome. A thin, tall patient with long fingers and a high arching palate is a giveaway for Marfan's. There is a high incidence of cardiac and aortic abnormalities associated with Marfanoid patients. Of special interest is an aortic aneurysm because of the connective tissue disorder.

Another characteristic appearance is seen in tertiary syphilis, often with an obvious nasal deformity. These patients as well have a high risk of abdominal aortic aneurysm.

Inspect the neck of the patient or any abnormal pulsations. A pulsatile mass along the course of the carotid artery may be an aneurysm. A pulsatile mass near the carotid bifurcation can be a carotid body tumor. Visible pulsations in the supraclavicular area are most commonly due to a tortuous subclavian artery; however, a subclavian artery aneurysm needs to be ruled out.

A rare phenomenon is to observe prominent collateral arterial pulsations in the upper torso in young adults, and this is typical of patients with *coarctation of aorta*.

Look for any clusters of blood vessels on any part of the body, particularly the extremities, as these may be arteriovenous malformations. Note if there is disparity in the growth of extremities, which is often associated with arteriovenous malformation. The side with the malformation tends to grow larger.

In thin individuals with a scaphoid abdomen, an abdominal aortic aneurysm may be visible as a pulsatile swelling in the midabdomen. Inspection of both groins and the popliteal spaces should be routine, looking for any visible pulsatile masses.

Visible Signs of Arterial Insufficiency

Next, look at the lower extremities for evidence of arterial disease. When you are examining the patient in a recumbent position, the feet might look normal in color. Ask the patient to elevate the extremity, and watch for any color change. If there is pallor of the elevated feet, it indicates abnormal circulation. Similarly, ask the patient to sit up on the edge of the bed, and again note if patient develops dependent rubor of the feet. One needs to make a clear distinction between dependent rubor and reactive hyperemia. The dependent rubor has a cyanotic tinge to the pinkness of the feet as a result of methemoglobin, whereas reactive hyperemia is just pink.

In a male (PAD is more common in men), absence of hair from the extremity with smooth, shiny skin will be an indicator of vascular insufficiency. Examine the nails closely. Nails tend to be brittle and deformed in patients with arterial insufficiency.

Discoloration

Look for discoloration of the toes, feet, or the entire extremity. A cyanotic extremity is often mistaken for acute ischemia. An acutely ischemic extremity is pale; remember the six Ps of acute arterial ischemia (pallor, pulselessness, pain, paralysis, paraesthesia, and poikilothermia). When a toe, multiple toes, or an extremity is cyanotic, it is important to note if the cyanosis will blanch or if the cyanosis is fixed. A blanching cyanosis is usually seen in patients with vasospastic disorders or in patients with venous outflow obstruction. A fixed cyanosis is an ominous sign and generally indicates nonviability of tissues. Occasionally one would see arterial insufficiency cause blanching cyanosis as in the case of a blue-toe syndrome. This is almost always secondary to an arterial embolic event to a toe. Sometimes microemboli originating in a plaque in the proximal arterial tree can produce very subtle findings on inspection. These microemboli, which might appear as tiny blue or purple dots on the tips of toes, can be easily overlooked on a cursory examination.

Ulceration

By definition, an ulcer is a breach in the continuity of an epithelial surface. Arterial ulcers tend to occur commonly over pressure points. They can be anywhere on the toes, foot, ankle, or lower leg. The arterial ulcers have certain features that distinguish them from other causes of ulcers. Typically, the arterial ulcer is described as a punched-out ulcer, which means they have a sharp, clear border, as if someone punched out cleanly a portion of skin and subcutaneous tissue from the center of it. These ulcers often have a necrotic base and do not show any signs of healing. As these ulcers are the result of deficient blood flow to the area, there is no zone of redness around them, on the contrary, they have pallor surrounding them. Arterial ulcers tend to be excruciatingly painful unless the patient is a diabetic with neuropathy. Pay attention to the depth of the ulcer as deep ulcers may have bone involvement with osteomyelitis.

Gangrene

Gangrene is defined as death of a part with superadded putrefaction to distinguish it from necrosis, which is simply death of a part. Gangrene may be dry or wet, and it is quite obvious which it is just on inspection.

Dry gangrene looks dry as the name implies, and there is generally a well-defined line of demarcation between the black leathery tissue and the viable pink tissue. If the dry gangrene involves a toe, the toe looks shriveled up.

Wet gangrene (also called moist gangrene), on the other hand, not only shows the black dead tissue but also shows redness, swelling, and drainage from the area. Often there is no clear line of demarcation in the wet gangrene, and it will not be unusual to have

81

accompanying crepitus in the soft tissue. Wet gangrene is a surgical emergency.

Gangrene, ulceration, and rest pain are all considered limb threatening.

Palpation

A complete vascular exam includes palpation of all arterial pulses, from superficial temporal artery on both temples to the pedal pulses in the feet.

Presence of superficial temporal pulse gives some assurance that the external carotid artery is patent. Examine the carotid artery pulses just anterior to the anterior border of the sternocleidomastoid muscle. The landmark for the carotid bifurcation is the level of the thyroid cartilage. In a slender neck, it is possible to feel the carotid bulb and any abnormality of it—for example, a carotid body tumor. A rare instance of a carotid artery aneurysm can also be easily felt on physical examination. Gently apply upward pressure on the cricoids cartilage, and feel for any downward movement with every systole. Presence of the downward movement is called tracheal tug, and this indicates an aneurysm of the arch of the aorta.

Palpation of the supraclavicular area will feel the subclavian arterial pulse in a number of patients as tortuosity of this vessel is quite common. After the subclavian artery palpation, one would move to the brachial, radial, and ulnar artery pulses. One would not normally feel for the axillary pulse unless the brachial pulse is absent.

At the wrist, both the radial and ulnar artery pulses should be felt. Remember that the dominant blood supply to the hand is from the ulnar artery. An Allen test should be performed if the patient is to undergo a puncture, cannulation, or harvest of the radial artery.

Allen Test

An Allen test is performed to check adequacy of blood flow to the hand via the ulnar artery. The patient is asked to elevate the hand to be tested and is asked to clench the fist. Apply pressure at the wrist to occlude both the radial and the ulnar pulses. Ask the patient to open the hand, and observe severe pallor of the hand. Next, release pressure over the ulnar artery, and observe the hand pink up almost instantaneously. It usually takes less than five to seven seconds for the hand to pink up, reassuring that there is adequate blood flow to the hand via the ulnar artery and it is the dominant vessel.

Palpate the abdomen for any pulsatile abdominal masses. Beware, not all pulsatile masses in the abdomen are aortic aneurysms. Any mass sitting on the abdominal aorta is likely to transmit aortic pulsations to the mass. An example would be a midtransverse colon mass presenting as a pulsating abdominal mass. So how does one clinically distinguish that from an abdominal aortic aneurysm? Today's medical student would say "Get an ultrasound" without realizing that he/she could make the diagnosis at the bedside instantaneously without any cost. The student needs to learn the difference between what is a transmitted pulsation versus what would be an expansile pulsation of an aneurysm. Place two fingers, the index finger of each hand separated by about an inch over the pulsating mass and observe. If the two fingers move just up and down with the pulsations, you can be sure that these are transmitted pulsations. If the two fingers go not only up and down but also away from each other, that is a classic sign of expansile pulsations from an aneurysm.

The same methodology can be applied to correct a very common mistake made in physical diagnosis of a small pulsatile mass at the wrist involving the radial artery. Commonly mistaken as radial artery aneurysms, these are usually ganglion of the wrist overlying the radial artery. The mass is too small to place two fingers on it as in AAA, so you pinch it gently between the index finger and thumb of the same hand. An aneurysm will separate the thumb from the index finger with each pulsation, whereas a ganglion will not.

Proceed with the remaining pulse palpation in the groins for femoral arteries, in the popliteal spaces for popliteal arteries, and the feet for dorsalis pedis and posterior tibial arteries. The popliteal pulses are difficult to feel unless you bend the knee slightly over both your hands. A very prominent or easily felt popliteal pulse should make one suspicious of a popliteal artery aneurysm.

Checking for skin temperature is a useful tool. Temperature of one extremity cooler than the other will signify a pathologic change. If both or all extremities are cool, it may be the effect of outside temperatures, or it may be seen in vasospastic disorders. Skin temperature is a very good marker for checking a revascularized limb.

Palpation is also used to feel for thrills, indicating either a stenosis of a major artery or a communication between an artery and a vein. The classic description of a thrill is likened to purring of a cat. An arterial stenosis producing turbulence of blood flow generates a thrill. The thrill is also generated when high-pressure arterial blood flows into a low-pressure vein as in an arteriovenous fistula. The arteriovenous fistula may be congenital or created for hemodialysis.

It is important to know that if the systemic blood pressure is low, the thrill disappears.

Checking for sensation and motor function would complete the palpation part of the exam. This exam is important under two sets of circumstances. It is valuable in evaluating patients with acute ischemia who would lose their sensation before motor function, and in patients with diabetes mellitus, lack of sensation confirms diabetic neuropathy. In patients with severe chronic ischemia, it may not be unusual to find peroneal nerve palsy presenting as a foot drop.

Auscultation

Auscultation of the arterial system is used to measure blood pressure, detect bruits and pericardial and pleural rubs, and make a distinction between a transmitted cardiac murmur and a bruit.

Start the auscultation by examining the carotid artery first. Listen at the carotid bifurcation located at the level of the thyroid cartilage. This is where it is easy to make the mistake of calling a transmitted cardiac murmur as a carotid bruit. The distinguishing feature is the pitch of the sound and the location. A carotid bruit will get higher pitched as you move from the supraclavicular area to the carotid bifurcation, and the cardiac murmur will be just the reverse. The murmur will get louder as you move away from the carotid bifurcation toward the heart. Sometimes this change is quite subtle, and even the best of clinicians can make a mistake.

Measure blood pressure in both arms, and note that it is more common to have lower blood pressure in the left arm because of a higher incidence of subclavian stenosis on the left. If there is a pressure differential between the two sides, the higher pressure is the correct one. In cases of significant arterial stenosis, it may not be possible to obtain a blood pressure with a stethoscope, and in that case, a Doppler may have to be used to measure at least the systolic blood pressure. Upon listening with a stethoscope just below the outer third of the clavicle, one might hear a bruit related to subclavian artery stenosis.

Listening in the precordial area might be fruitful in detecting a pericardial rub, a sign of pericarditis.

Auscultation of the lung bases can be productive in picking up a pleural friction rub as seen sometimes in pulmonary emboli.

Auscultation of the abdomen comes next. Listening for abdominal bruits will be a helpful aid in the diagnosis of renovascular hypertension, mesenteric ischemia, and aortoiliac occlusive disease. The location of the bruit and its intensity are the features to look for. Renal artery bruits are located more toward the flanks, whereas mesenteric and aortic occlusive bruits are more centrally located in the epigastrium. Bruits in the lower quadrants are associated with iliac artery occlusive disease.

Bruits in the groins are associated with femoral artery stenosis. Auscultation of the arterial system generally ends in the groins as it is not common to find bruits lower down in the extremities. The only exception to this is an arteriovenous fistula or malformation where presence of a bruit will confirm an arterial component.

BEDSIDE EXAMINATION OF THE ARTERIAL SYSTEM WITH A DOPPLER ULTRASOUND

In the twenty-first century, physical examination of the arterial system includes a bedside evaluation of the circulation using a handheld Doppler ultrasound. The use of Doppler ultrasound gives information on three important aspects of the arterial system. First and foremost, one can establish presence or absence of blood flow, as feeling for presence or absence of pulses is a crude and unreliable method of examination. Second, once you hear blood flow, you can evaluate the quality of blood flow by remarking on whether it is triphasic (normal), biphasic, or monophasic (abnormal). Last, one can quantify the blood flow by measuring segmental pressures. Though measuring thigh pressure, calf pressure, and ankle pressure will give a more complete picture, it is generally left for the noninvasive vascular lab to do those measurements. A quick bedside evaluation can be done by just recording the ankle pressure and then calculating the ankle-brachial index (ABI) for quantifying the blood flow. It should be known that this evaluation is not suitable for a diabetic because their arteries may be noncompressible and will give a falsely elevated ABI.

When the pedal pulses are absent and we suspect an occlusion of the superficial femoral artery, it is possible to evaluate the collateral circulation via profunda femoris artery to substantiate the ABI value. This is accomplished by measuring a cuff blood pressure just above the knee and also just below the knee, and the ratio between the two pressures is referred to as the profunda popliteal index (PPI). This value complements the recorded ABI and is helpful in formulating a treatment plan.

VENOUS SYSTEM

Examination of the venous system consists of examination of the superficial venous system and the deep venous system. The general theme of inspecting, palpating, percussing, and auscultating can be applied to the venous system as well. The examination is not limited to just extremities as venous abnormalities may be seen anywhere on the body. Be reminded that of all the various systems in the body, the venous system has the highest incidence of anatomical variations.

SUPERFICIAL VENOUS SYSTEM

Inspection

In majority of cases, it is the lower extremity that will exhibit abnormalities of the superficial venous system; however, a keen eye should look at the patient from head to toes. One of the abnormalities seen more often in locations other than lower legs is venous malformations presenting as clusters of veins in an area. If one notes these on the upper extremity with accompanying disparity of limb growth on that side, it is likely to be an arteriovenous malformation. There is an exception to this in the lower extremity of a patient with a Klippel-Trenaunay syndrome (limb overgrowth with venous malformation without an arterial component).

Any coursing superficial veins around the shoulder girdle, hip, or anterior abdominal wall are usually collateral veins secondary to occlusion of the deep system. Venous cluster around the umbilicus (caput medusae) in patients with portal hypertension has been mentioned earlier in the text.

Directing attention to the lower extremities, look for presence of superficial varicose veins. If varicose veins are present, note if their distribution is along the medial aspect of the thigh and leg, which would indicate varicosities of the greater saphenous system, or posterior lower leg, which points to varicosities of the lesser saphenous system. If the varicose veins are scattered between these two locations, they are most likely tributaries of the greater or lesser saphenous systems. A well-recognized superficial vein that connects the lesser saphenous vein to the greater saphenous vein is known as vein of *Giacomini*. This vein runs posteromedially from the greater saphenous to connect with the lesser saphenous. Visually follow the course of greater saphenous vein. An easily visible raised erythematous cluster of painful veins along the course of the greater saphenous is classic superficial phlebitis.

Carefully look at the skin of the lower extremities for any breach of the epithelium (ulcer), any discoloration, presence of any scars particularly in the *gaiter area* (medial lower one-third of the leg), or any visible evidence of *lipodermatosclerosis* (described often as an inverted-champagne-bottle appearance). Look for any small unimpressive venule slightly raised above the surface of the skin and sometimes scabbed over. Beware of this finding as these are potential spontaneously rupturing veins, and they tend to bleed like an artery because of very high venous pressure.

The brownish discoloration of the lower extremities from chronic venous stasis is from deposition of hemosiderin pigment in the skin. Hemosiderin is a by-product of red cell breakdown, which is then taken up by macrophages. Most of the time, this discoloration of chronic venous disease is permanent and will not fade from the lower extremity as opposed to the hemosiderin that stains the skin from bleeding into tissues, which would eventually disappear. In some patients with chronic venous stasis, this discoloration is so dark that the legs look almost black.

Another abnormality of the skin seen on inspection is a rash with an angry look or weeping from the leg. In patients with venous disease, this is generally from what is referred to as *stasis dermatitis*. There are different degrees of severity of this ailment, and in its severe form, it can be quite disabling.

Ulceration secondary to venous disease is distinctively different from arterial ulcers. Venous ulcers are generally seen in the *gaiter area* and tend to be irregular in shape. This is in contrast to the arterial ulcers that are sharply defined with punched-out borders. The table below shows some of the distinguishing features of both arterial and venous ulcers.

Table: Arterial and Venous Ulcers Compared

Type of ulcer	Location	Margins	Ulcer bed	Granulation tissue	Surrounding skin	Associated with
ARTERIAL	Anywhere, particularly bony prominences	Clean and punched out	Necrotic and sloughy and deep	Absent	Pale	Loss of hair and brittle dystrophic nails
VENOUS	Distal 1/3 of leg medially (gaiter area)	Irregular because of attempts at healing	Shallow and often pink	Present	Zone of hyperemia	Hemosiderin pigmentation or stasis dermatitis

The venous ulcers tend to be quite painful. The arterial ulcers in a nondiabetic patient may be associated with rest pain, but in diabetics, the ulcers will be painless because of diabetic neuropathy. One should keep this in mind if a patient with venous ulcers happens to have diabetic neuropathy.

Though venous ulcers are most common in the *gaiter area* medially, a patient with chronic venous stasis may present with an ulcer anterior, lateral, or posterior parts of the leg. These ulcers will often result from trauma and will not be spontaneous.

Palpation

Palpation of the superficial venous system can be used to determine the direction of venous blood flow in the superficial vein. For example, if some prominent veins are seen on the chest wall, fingers from one hand can be used to apply pressure to occlude the vein, while a finger from the other hand presses blood out of a segment of the vein and holds pressure on the other end of the segment. By releasing one finger at a time, the direction of blood refilling the vein can be easily determined. If one suspects occlusion of a major vein, the direction of flow in the superficial vein will be away from that major vein. This method can be used on any of the superficial collateral veins or superficial lower extremity veins. In the lower extremity, reversal of venous flow usually indicates incompetence of the vein.

Palpation of a raised erythematous cluster of veins, which feel hard and tender, is typical of superficial thrombophlebitis.

Sometimes, small hard nodules are palpated in the veins of the upper or lower extremity. A relatively common cause of those nodules in the upper extremity is organized thrombi from intravenous administration of drugs. A rare cause of these nodules in upper or lower extremity is a *phlebolith*. These are calcification within the vein, forming a small stone. These are more common in the pelvic veins but can be seen outside the pelvis once in a while.

The use of a Doppler ultrasound for bedside evaluation of the venous system and the more sophisticated duplex imaging in the vascular lab has some classical tests for venous testing sidelined. For the sake of being complete and to have an alternative to the modern technology, a student of surgery should be familiar with these tests and should also know how to perform them.

Trendelenburg Test

This test was done to check the competence of the superficial venous system. The patient is asked to lie down flat. The lower limb in question is raised to empty the superficial veins, and then a tourniquet is placed at the saphenofemoral junction, just tight enough to occlude the superficial and not the deep system. The patient is then asked to stand up and watch carefully how the superficial veins fill from below—upward, slowly. Remove the tourniquet, and observe if the veins suddenly fill very quickly, and if this happens, it clearly indicates incompetence of the superficial veins, allowing the veins to fill from above, downward. If the removal of tourniquet does not make a difference, it can be inferred that the superficial saphenous vein is competent. By placing the tourniquet at different levels on the leg, a segment of an incompetent vein can be detected.

Perthes Test

This test determines patency of the deep venous system. Again, the patient is asked to lie down, and the leg is raised to empty the venous blood, and a tourniquet is placed at the saphenofemoral junction, like in the test above. The patient is then asked to get up and walk around in the examining room. If the patient can do that comfortably and there are no changes noted in the veins of the leg, the test is negative, indicating patency of the deep system and normal venous outflow. However, as the patient starts to walk around, if he/she feels pressure and, later, pain in the leg, and the veins in that leg stand out more than before, then it will mean a positive test indicating occlusion of the deep system.

BEDSIDE EXAMINATION OF THE VENOUS SYSTEM WITH A DOPPLER ULTRASOUND

Bedside examination of the venous system with a Doppler ultrasound certainly complements the clinical examination. The Doppler ultrasound can not only detect the presence of an occlusive thrombus in the venous system but also localize the occlusive thrombus; however, its accuracy could not be relied upon. It is a well-accepted fact that clinical diagnosis of DVT is only 50 percent accurate, and in my opinion, adding a bedside Doppler exam adds at least another 10 percent to the accuracy of diagnosis of DVT, thus making it better than the toss of a coin.

Venous examination with a Doppler requires one to develop a certain discipline in first localizing a vein and then learning to concentrate on the sounds of venous blood flow and ignoring the sounds of an adjacent pulsatile artery. The best location to learn and familiarize oneself with this technique is the femoral region. The femoral artery is easily located with a Doppler, and just medial to it is the femoral vein. Upon listening to the sound of the flow in the femoral vein, it is noted that the venous flow changes with inspiration and expiration. With inspiration, there is a reduction of venous return as the diaphragm moves down, and increasing the intra-abdominal pressure impedes venous return. As the patient breathes out, with expiration, a negative pressure is created in the thoracic cage and venous return is enhanced. These changes in the venous flow with the respiratory excursions can be easily appreciated by listening to the femoral vein with a Doppler. Absence of these variations in the venous flow with breathing indirectly implies an obstruction to venous flow between where the Doppler probe is and the chest, whereas crisp and clear venous flow sounds that vary with inhaling and exhaling indicate unobstructed flow between the Doppler probe and the chest.

Leaving the Doppler probe on the femoral vein and listening to the venous flow, squeeze the leg near the ankle, and you will hear a loud sound from a column of blood getting squeezed past the Doppler probe. This transient sound is produced by augmentation of venous blood flow with squeezing and is sometimes referred to as the "A" sound. When one hears this clear, crisp sound by squeezing the ankle, it implies that there is no obstruction to transmission of this sound from the ankle to the groin, and it is unlikely that an occlusive thrombus is present between those two points. If the sound is not transmitted from the ankle to the groin, by moving the Doppler probe to the popliteal vein, an area of obstruction can be localized.

If there is no clinical history to suspect a diagnosis of DVT, learning to use the Doppler will avoid a lot of unnecessary imaging tests.

SUMMARY AND CONCLUSION

It has been clearly pointed out in this manuscript that a detailed history of a patient's illness and a thorough physical examination should get the examiner much closer to the diagnosis without the many tests ordered as routine in today's practice of medicine. Keeping an inquisitive and an analytical mind to put the symptoms and physical findings together to arrive at a diagnosis should be taught to every student of surgery or medicine.

When the examiner orders any blood tests or imaging studies for a patient, he/she should pose a question to himself/herself. Is this test or imaging study useful and necessary to make the diagnosis, and is this going to change the treatment plan in any way? If the answer to this question is yes, then the test and studies were justified. But if the answer is negative, the tests and studies were unnecessary and were probably ordered because of insecurity and fear of litigation.

One cannot practice good medicine under the constant fear of litigation (defensive medicine), which would normally lead to substandard care and add tremendously to the cost of care without improving the outcomes.

In my opinion, the solid foundation of basics of good history taking and a careful thorough physical examination can significantly improve the quality of care and at the same time reduce the cost of care. Judicious use of your ears to listen to the complaints, your mind to analyze the symptoms, your trained hands to feel and palpate, and your stethoscope to listen to abnormal sounds will go a long way in making you a good clinician.